"The message of psychoanalysis, masterfully voiced by Sergio Aguilar, goes against the grain of our psychologized, almost zoological 'self(ie) understanding', the latter perfectly attuned to neoliberal digitalized capitalism. Look into Aguilar's Lacanian mirror, and see another subject: alienated in its own image and body, always differing from what it says/is said to be. Behold that subject, 'necessarily presuppos[ing] the other': this perspective is indispensable for those who still believe in collective emancipation."

Jan De Vos, psychoanalytic theorist and author of amongst others *The Digitalisation of (Inter)Subjectivity* (Routledge, 2020)

"This book is both a rigorous reprise and a creative subversion of Lacan's mirror scene. With *A Contemporary Return to the Lacanian Mirror*, Aguilar shows how the contemporary subject, far from forming a unified coherence, is fragmented, captured, and re-performed through the selfie, the neoliberal marketplace of identities, and the illusions of imaginary autonomy: to read this book is to realize that Lacan's mirror was always an abyss. It is a rare work, in dialogue with Freud, Lacan, and cultural studies, but also with the most current avatars of technology and desire. An essential reading for libidinal Marxists, media scholars, and political psychoanalysts alike."

Carlos Gómez Camarena, Psychoanalyst and Researcher, Forums of the Lacanian Field / Universidad Iberoamericana, Mexico

A CONTEMPORARY RETURN TO THE LACANIAN MIRROR

A Contemporary Return to the Lacanian Mirror is a discussion on *The Mirror Stage as Formative of the I Function as Revealed in Psychoanalytic Experience*, a capital text within Lacanian thought and psychoanalytic history.

Drawing on Freudian and Lacanian concepts, Sergio J. Aguilar Alcalá explores the consequences of the mirror stage for human subjectivity: an alienation of any remains of animal nature, an aggressive drive at the heart of our relationship to others and to ourselves, and an introjection of the desire of the other as our own desire. These consequences allow for a critique of, among other things, the test zoologists use to 'prove' that animals can recognize themselves in the mirror, the notions of 'freedom' and 'agency' that mainstream communication and media studies ascribe to selfies on social media, and the neoliberal uses of labor psychology and identity politics to flatten the intricacies and contradictions within our/selves. The book begins with consideration of the imago and identification, then discusses the consequences of Lacan's three crossroads for our conception of human subjectivity. Aguilar Alcalá concludes by discussing how the Lacanian mirror stage enables us to go beyond the Imaginary traps provoked by today's media and cultural landscape, using the aphorism mentioned at the end of the mirror stage text: thou art that.

A Contemporary Return to the Lacanian Mirror will be of great interest to academics and scholars of psychoanalytic studies, communication and media studies. It will also appeal to those working within the humanities and specifically in the philosophy of the human–animal relationship, images in digital culture and critical theory.

Sergio J. Aguilar Alcalá practices psychoanalysis in Mexico and has published several works at the intersections of psychoanalysis, communication theory and film studies. Contact: sergio.aguilaralcala@gmail.com

THE LINES OF THE SYMBOLIC IN PSYCHOANALYSIS SERIES

Series Editor: Ian Parker, Manchester Psychoanalytic Matrix

Psychoanalytic clinical and theoretical work is always embedded in specific linguistic and cultural contexts and carries their traces, traces which this series attends to in its focus on multiple contradictory and antagonistic 'lines of the Symbolic'. This series takes its cue from Lacan's psychoanalytic work on three registers of human experience, the Symbolic, the Imaginary and the Real, and employs this distinctive understanding of cultural, communication and embodiment to link with other traditions of cultural, clinical and theoretical practice beyond the Lacanian symbolic universe. The Lines of the Symbolic in Psychoanalysis Series provides a reflexive reworking of theoretical and practical issues, translating psychoanalytic writing from different contexts, grounding that work in the specific histories and politics that provide the conditions of possibility for its descriptions and interventions to function. The series makes connections between different cultural and disciplinary sites in which psychoanalysis operates, questioning the idea that there could be one single correct reading and application of Lacan. Its authors trace their own path, their own line through the Symbolic, situating psychoanalysis in relation to debates which intersect with Lacanian work, explicating it, extending it and challenging it.

Queer Theory, Lacanian Psychoanalysis, Sexual Politics
From Norm to Desire
Luiz Valle Junior

Taking Back Desire: A Psychoanalytic Approach to Queerness and Neoliberalism on Screen
James Lawrence Slattery

On the Theory and Clinic of Lacanian Psychoanalysis: Speaking of Lacan
Chris Vanderwees

Queer Psychoanalysis: Minor Clinic and Deconstruction of Gender
Fabrice Bourlez

A Contemporary Return to the Lacanian Mirror: You Are That
Sergio J. Aguilar Alcalá

For more information about the series, please visit: https://www.routledge.com/The-Lines-of-the-Symbolic-in-Psychoanalysis-Series/book-series/KARNLOS

A CONTEMPORARY RETURN TO THE LACANIAN MIRROR

You Are That

Sergio J. Aguilar Alcalá

Routledge
Taylor & Francis Group
LONDON AND NEW YORK

Designed cover image: Getty

First published 2026
by Routledge
4 Park Square, Milton Park, Abingdon, Oxon OX14 4RN

and by Routledge
605 Third Avenue, New York, NY 10158

Routledge is an imprint of the Taylor & Francis Group, an informa business

British Library Cataloguing in Publication Data
A catalogue record for this book is available from the British Library

Library of Congress Cataloging-in-Publication Data
A catalog record has been requested for this book

ISBN: 9781041074687 (hbk)
ISBN: 9781041074663 (pbk)
ISBN: 9781003640653 (ebk)

DOI: 10.4324/9781003640653

Typeset in Times New Roman
by Taylor & Francis Books

CONTENTS

SERIES PREFACE FOR SERGIO J. AGUILAR ALCALÁ'S *A CONTEMPORARY RETURN TO THE LACANIAN MIRROR: YOU ARE THAT*

A problem that bedevils Lacanian psychoanalytic theory, and not only Lacanian, is that the author and reader confront the text as if it were a mirror, anxious to find confirmation that what they thought Lacan said can be found there, anxious to find confirmation that their own singular take is correct. This book confronts us with the mirroring process and throws back to us some uncomfortable unsettling thoughts about what it is to be human and, for that matter, what it is to be another animal among all the others we still share our planet with.

The problem is acute in the clinic, and the analyst has the task of disentangling their own mirrored understanding of what is going on, including what they might believe their analysand is saying, thinking even, from the actual flow of the words, the narrative that the analysand constructs in the session. That is, there must be a careful attention to what is Imaginary—that which is reflected back to the analyst from the assumptions they have already made about what they hear—from the Symbolic domain in which the analysand travels and configures themselves as a subject in their own speech.

Against these two registers, Imaginary and Symbolic, there is the third register of the Real, that which hits us in the face, in the guts, refuses to budge, insists on its presence. You will find each of these three registers, sometimes teased apart and sometimes tangled together, in this strange book on the mirror and identity in Lacanian communication and social theory.

In the domain of social theory, Lacanian psychoanalysis sometimes flowers, to good and bad effect, with consequences that run far beyond its own specific clinical domain, the domain that Lacan himself addressed in his Seminars. Here is a book that takes that risk, venturing into political judgements that the reader will need to attend to, and will need to sift out of what is of their own position, what is actually being claimed and what is being mirrored back to them by the author.

What is sometimes forgotten in some of the hardline Symbolic-focused representations of Lacanian psychoanalysis is that the realm of the Imaginary is also essential for communication, for a sense of connection to others and for self-understanding. The Lacanian psychoanalyst does not ignore the Imaginary, but attends to it, handles it carefully, respecting the many ways in which analysands bring strange forms of speech into the clinic, forms of speech to which they are attached, that have deep implications for their own subjectivity.

When the Lacanian psychoanalyst ventures into the public domain, beyond the clinic, it is not simply to dispel Imaginary and Symbolic conceptions of identity, but to explore how these conceptions function to separate people from each other, and sometimes also to draw people together, enable them to find common cause. Conceptions of identity at the level of the Imaginary and the Symbolic are mobilized in contexts of pain at exclusion and in attempts to find individual and collective ways of being in the world. Mirrors are themselves also, Lacan showed us, structured materially and symbolically, both as defences against and sometimes engagements with the Real.

Psychoanalytic clinical and theoretical work circulates through multiple intersecting antagonistic symbolic universes. This series opens connections between different cultural sites in which Lacanian work has developed in distinctive ways, in forms of work that question the idea that there could be a single correct reading and application. The Lines of the Symbolic in Psychoanalysis series provides a reflexive reworking of psychoanalysis that transmits Lacanian writing from around the world, steering a course between the temptations of a metalanguage and imaginary reduction, between the claim to provide a god's eye view of psychoanalysis and the idea that psychoanalysis must everywhere be the same. And the elaboration of psychoanalysis in the symbolic here grounds its theory and practice in the history and politics of the work in a variety of interventions that touch the real.

Ian Parker
Manchester Psychoanalytic Matrix

ACKNOWLEDGMENTS

Although I can think of many anecdotes and people who, indirectly, caused this book, I think it would be better (at least shorter) to mention only those who were directly involved.

First and foremost, I want to thank those people, many of whom I don't know by name, whose questions, discussions, suggestions, complaints and flatteries, while attending the many lectures, conferences and classes I've given on the topics of this book (and others), have greatly improved the correction, rectification, strengthening and transmission of my ideas. These people also include colleagues, professors and friends. I want to thank, particularly in this respect, Vicente Castellanos Cerda, for his honest and warm support, encouragement, reviewing and questioning.

Second, I want to thank the moral supporters who also enabled and encouraged me to pursue the completion of this book. In particular, Meryvid Pérez, Carlos Gómez Camarena and Luca.

And last, but not least: thanks to those who listen.

FOREWORD

Ours is the age of identity. Never have we been more concerned with representation, with recognition, with the need to 'feel seen' and with the need to express ourselves in positive terms. Whichever side of the debate around 'identity politics' we might be on, we can't hide from the fact that identity is expressed wherever we look. The psychoanalyst Jacques Lacan also considered identity to be the cornerstone of social and cultural life, but in a way that runs quite counter to the dominant discourses of identity that dominate society today.

The starting point for Aguilar's text is to follow a central maxim of Lacan: the idea of locating identification "at the very heart of the birth of subjectivity." So far, so good: identity is critical to the formation of the subject, and therefore it should concern us greatly. But Lacan's important insight would make another turn of the screw. As Aguilar puts it, he would insist "that the very idea of the Self only arises through the other."

In other words, the first moment of identity is the first moment of society, where we come to see ourselves as a being in the (social) world through the (mis)recognition of the other, and of the other's (mis)recognition of ourselves. There is no identity without society, and without the particular manifestation of society into which each of us is uniquely welcomed at the point of our formation as a subject. The idea that society gets in the way of us being ourselves, therefore, is flawed to its core. Here is where much contemporary thinking goes wrong, and why Freud and Lacan can be redeemed or returned to with particular force today.

This critical moment of the subject's identity formation and simultaneous entry into society was famously visualized in the image of a toddler first looking at itself in the mirror. It would come to be called 'the mirror stage,' and the essay first containing the idea would go on to be the most well-known of Lacan's texts, studied often on literature degrees, in film studies and even occasionally in psychology and philosophy. Over the years, the concept has been bullet-pointed and summarized and passed down in a nearly packaged form (it has become a received idea) so often as to have lost much of its critical importance and contribution. That is, until Aguilar's book.

In that essay on the mirror stage, Lacan would argue that the moment of looking into the mirror constitutes the creation of "the armour of an alienating identity" taken on by the subject, so that at the very moment that the subject becomes a subject, protected from the world by their identity, they are also alienated from their image of themselves. To enter culture, the little human being pays a price. From that moment on, they become a lacking, failed subject who can never live up to their own image of themselves. The cost of entry to the social order—no matter who you are—is an infinite alienation from others and from oneself. For Lacan, the subject lives from that moment on, tarrying with a gap at the core of subjectivity, until death.

Aguilar traces the root of this idea to Freud and even further, focusing on the fact that for this identity-formation process to take place, the subject cannot be alone but can only exist through their relationship to the other. In 1895, inspired by his recent collaboration with Joseph Breuer, Freud had begun to draft a document never published during his lifetime, which was discovered posthumously and which we know today as *Project for a Scientific Psychology*. There, he writes that "it is in relation to a fellow human-being that a human-being learns to cognize" (Freud, 1966/I, p. 331). For Aguilar, here:

> Freud has just realized, via the pleasure–displeasure relation, *how fundamental the other is for the constitution of the ego*: the ego is constituted through *cognizing* the other, to discern the other from the self, a matter that, later in his work, Freud understood as *identification*.

It is "through this pleasure–displeasure system [that] the ego manages to create a relation of communication between itself and the world." The moment of identification is the moment in which the subject begins to communicate with others and with the world.

In this sense, the model of subjectivity proposed here might be said to constitute a significant break from—and attack on—the commoditized subjects of digital capitalism. Those subjects are marked by the promise of fulfilment, the denial of lack and the fantasy of completion. These subjects reach for closure and representation as if it is possible, rather than accepting its inevitable failure. Aguilar is perhaps influenced by the Slovene School of Psychoanalysis in this regard. Mladen Dolar has made a point of establishing a difference between the approach of the Ljubljana School of psychoanalysis and that of Louis Althusser. In short, the Althusserian approach, and some of the Marxist traditions which followed it, insisted on alienation as a condition that needed overcoming. This—the Ljubljana psychoanalysts would argue—falls into a utopian trap: for these thinkers, individuality that is not alienated is—at least in theory—possible.

A properly psychoanalytic approach—as conceived by Freud, Lacan and Aguilar—is to accept the inevitable alienation of the subject, and perhaps even see in it the potential for a locus of connection between all subjects, no matter how diverse and particular. In other words, from its multiplicity of differences and particularisms comes a universalism—a universalism of lack and alienation. This is what tends to be forgotten in social life today—and Aguilar discusses everything from film to new media to the culture of selfies—leading to positivist and completist conceptions of identity that lead us to think of ourselves as individuals who can exist without each other. For Aguilar:

> The mirror stage allows Lacan to characterize human subjectivity, in "socially elaborated situations," via three main consequences vectors: (1) it is mediated by the desire of the other, (2) it mutates rivalry with the other into objects, and (3) it places the subject in a position alienated from any natural process.

These three pillars of identity and identification guide Aguliar's reading, and he proposes, ultimately, that much of the identitarian discourses of the present—including and sometimes especially those which present themselves as progressive and liberal—ignore these features of identity.

Among other things, the book playfully considers mirrors and animals, starting with an experiment conducted with dolphins to see if they can recognize themselves in a mirror. The dolphins seemed to display self-consciousness by noting marks placed on their bodies that they could only see in the mirror. Lacan and Freud were obsessed with animals, from rats to sardines to horses and elephants, and the question of what constitutes humanity is at the heart of this book as it was at the core of their work. Through this analysis, Aguilar argues that "what defines the human being is precisely its name, where we find the necessary doubleness to affirm itself: the human being is a continuous attempt to be a human." Like the toddler looking in the mirror, it wants to be the identity it perceives there. The difference between humans and animals is that "the human is inhabited by an irreducible gap between its body and its ego." For Aguilar, "the name for that gap is *subject*."

The subjectivity that arises from this gap is something present in us all. It is, in this sense, universal. Universality is unpopular today because it easily becomes a universalism in positive terms, which can be prescriptive and exclusionary. Particularisms are much easier to handle, and ours is a society that identifies us quickly and easily in particularist terms. But this approach fails because it functions only to emphasize our differences, rather than what we do have in common—the gap in subjectivity itself.

On the contrary, a psychoanalytic approach would be to accept the inevitable alienation of the subject and see in it the potential for a locus of connection between all subjects, no matter how diverse and particular. In other words, from its multiplicity of differences and particularisms comes a universalism—a universalism of lack and alienation, at the heart of what it means to be a human subject tarrying with its relationship to the world in a way that animals cannot.

In the two most hard-hitting chapters, Aguilar thoughtfully engages and critiques many of the now-normative discourses in neoliberal capitalism, including cancel culture, intersectionality and the politics of 'diversity.' He argues for the 'selfie' as a neoliberal weapon that encourages a certain conception of ourselves which lines up with what he calls the "sovereign self" of identity politics. This dominant conception of identity leads to "the separation from the other sustained in a 'self-enclosure of self-identified victims.'" Against these conceptions of identity that are embodied in the language of *diversity*, he argues for politics of *difference* which

> only recognizes identity in a point that disturbs the constitution of a totalizing identity: difference is not the difference between one and the other (that is a matter of diversity), but of conflict immanent to the establishment of that very diversity.

Aguilar's Lacanian approach, then, cuts strongly against the identitarian discourses of the moment.

This conception of identity as an immanent gap or conflict leads into Aguilar's class argument: that "it is impossible to include class struggle as an identity struggle" because "the class struggle is on the side of difference itself, because its resolution does not bet on a just coexistence between diverse classes: the only solution to the class struggle is the abolition of all classes." As such, class struggle would be against identities as we know them today—as they are understood even among progressives—and for the kind of universal subjectivity giving rise to conflict, difference and alienation that would necessitate the abolishment of identities as we know them.

Against a society that divides and particularizes, then, Aguilar offers us perhaps the ultimate hope—that since there is no subject without the other, and no identity without community and society, those attempts to separate us on the grounds of identity will necessarily fail, since identity is only possible in and through each other, only possible together.

Alfie Bown
King's College London

Reference

Freud, Sigmund. [1895] (1966). "Project for a Scientific Psychology." In *The Standard Edition of The Complete Psychological Works of Sigmund Freud*, Vol. I. The Hogarth Press, pp. 281–397.

1

INTRODUCTION

You are that Dolphin

Since the 1970s, there have been multiple experiments, with varied results, in which attempts have been made to determine whether animals recognize themselves when they are in front of a mirror. A famous one is that of Diane Reiss and Lori Marino (2001), in which they 'proved' that bottlenose dolphins (*Tursiops truncatus*) can recognize themselves in a mirror. The method was one that had already been tested in apes and other animals: a mark was placed on a part of the animal's body that it could not see unless it was in front of a mirror (on its face, or on a part of its abdomen).

The methodology of this experiment was to study the behavior of the dolphins at three moments: when a mark was placed on them, when a mark was *pretended to* be drawn (with a marker that was actually empty) and when *no* mark was placed on them. It was verified that when the dolphins *did* have the mark, they went to the mirror and spent *more* time in front of it than when they were *pretended* to be marked, and *more* time in this second instance than when they were *not* marked at all. In conclusion, the study states that the dolphins used the mirror to investigate parts of their body that had been marked: "These findings, therefore, offer the first convincing evidence that nonprimate species, the bottlenose dolphin, is capable of MSR [Mirror Self-Recognition]" (Reiss & Marino, 2001, p. 5942).

The conclusion of the experiment is that the dolphin recognizes its own body in the image that the mirror gives it, that it recognizes that this image is that of itself. Under this conception, the mirror image of one's own body offers the individual who looks at himself a kind of *container* of himself, a Gestalt image that becomes actual when we 'see ourselves' in the mirror, when we say 'that is me.' The image that the mirror gives me back is the one that allows me to verify my own body, an image that offers me an identity in which I verify myself. The mirror shows me what I am already made of, *what I am*.

DOI: 10.4324/9781003640653-1

Is this what Lacan means by the mirror stage? Is the mirror stage the promise of a completeness that the mirror offers for the subject to perceive itself 'as it is'?

Preliminary note on *The Mirror Stage*

Of all the Lacanian texts published in the *Écrits* in 1966, perhaps none has been more widely discussed outside psychoanalytic circles than the one entitled *The Mirror Stage as Formative of the* I *Function as Revealed in Psychoanalytic Experience* (for the rest of this book, I will abbreviate it as *The Mirror Stage*). Presented at the XVI International Congress of Psychoanalysis in 1949, and originating in a first version that was presented at the same Congress in 1936, Lacan proposes in this text his concept of "the mirror stage," which condenses some discussions that were taking place in psychoanalysis and psychology at the time (such as comparative psychology with animals and the contributions of the Gestalt school).

The Mirror Stage text has been reflected upon, quite deeply, in film studies, feminism, digital communication, humanities and philosophy. However, it is not my intention to offer a panoramic view of those discussions or critique them, which you can find in almost every introduction to Lacanian teaching. My intention is to present paths this *écrit* still has to offer for contemporary crossroads of psychoanalysis with psychology, communication theory, political discussions, animal philosophy, among other fields.

The title of the *écrit*, in addition to being extensive, contains something of importance when reading a translation and not the original French. In Lacan's language, there are two words for what in English could be used, in many cases, as the first person of the singular, "I." In French, there are "moi" and "je," and their difference is quite important in Lacan's work, and plays certain implications in the text. In French, the tonic pronoun *je* is used to denote the pronoun *I* whenever it is accompanied by a verb (*Je suis Lacan*, I am Lacan); whereas *moi*, functions as an atonic pronoun, similar to *me/mine* (*C'est à moi*, It is mine; *Avec moi*, With me).

The important point here is that, when Lacan speaks of *le Je*, we should not understand it as *the I* that speaks, but as a *function* that the I occupies. As will be expanded in this text, this supposes the existence of two egos for Lacan: the Imaginary ego, corresponding to the *imago* that the subject assumes and which we can qualify as *the ego of the individual who speaks*, and, on the other hand, the Symbolic Ego, which is a function *resulting from and condition for* assuming that *imago* and which we can qualify as *the Ego of the speaking subject*. As we can already see, individual and subject are not synonymous for Lacan.

The text *The Mirror Stage* will serve as an axis to introduce several fundamental concepts of Lacanian thought, which are usually grouped in what some call *the Lacan of the Imaginary*: the role of the *imago* and the other in the constitution of the I, the distinction between two "I" (*moi* and *je*, in French), the distinction between identity and identification, the split between the body and the I, the function of the I as an alienation of the subject, the distinction between the animal instinct and the alienated nature of the subject, the function of aggressiveness as constitutive of human subjectivity, and a first introduction to the relationship between the desire of the subject and the desire of the other.

Other Lacanian texts that will complement the exposition of the following chapters are *Beyond the* "Reality Principle" (1936), *Presentation on Psychical Causality* (1946), *Aggressiveness in Psychoanalysis* (1948), *A Theoretical Introduction to the Functions of Psychoanalysis in Criminology* (1950), *The Situation of Psychoanalysis and the Training of Psychoanalysts in 1956* (1956), *Remarks on Daniel Lagache's Presentation:* "Psychoanalysis and Personality Structure" (1960) and some elements from Seminar 1, 10 and 20, as well as contributions from critical psychology, zoology, articles on the *selfie*, studies of children's drawing, manuals on assertive communication and labor psychology.[1] This work intends to function as an argumentation on an essential key for understanding Lacanian work: the subject is the result of a fundamental alienation of the ego with the body, which does not allow any sense of identity completeness, but of continuous identifications that work with and for the other.

I will start with a brief discussion of Freud's concept of *identification*, restricted to some ideas found in 1895's *Project* (1966/I), 1912's *Papers on Technique* (1958/XII) and 1921's *Group Psychology and Analysis of the Ego* (1955/XVIII).[2] For reasons that will become evident in the following sections, the Freudian concept of *identification* is key, since it explicitly presents the way the subject relates to the other, and how this other supposes a way in which the subject itself is constituted.

Right after Freud, I will present a general overview of selected sections of the Lacanian *écrit*, emphasizing the paradoxical effect (splitting and reuniting) the imago has on the body and the ego, the traps the concept of identity brings when we confuse it with identification, the problem the human has when trying to 'assume' its body as its own and the theoretical consequences the mirror stage brings into Lacanian psychoanalysis.

The rest of the book discusses, in three chapters, the consequences of Lacan's three crossroads for our conception of human subjectivity in relation to the other (both the other person and society as a whole).

The first is the relationship we have with animals. This relationship is crucial in this epoch, at a time when humans are much more aware of the impact they have on the planet and its ecosystems, while at the same time being unable to take a stand in their fundamental difference towards animals: in popular discussions, humans are reduced to being 'just another animal,' while and animals are 'humanized' through social media and pop culture discourses we have for them. It's becoming quite common, in urban environments, to see dogs in strollers and infants in dog leashes. This 'hominization of nature' even infects the way zoologists think of animal behavior, as the problems we can see arising in the "Mirror Self-Recognition" tests they use to (so they claim) prove that an animal recognizes itself.

The second crossroads is the location of the aggressivity towards others as a fundamental feature of the constitution of human subjectivity due to the split between image and imago. In today's social media landscape, the pictures known as *selfies* evoke a particular instance to show 'our' image. At the same time, we disown our images—that is, the selfie is a paradoxical image where we show ourselves by the act of losing ourselves in favor of the other's desire. This act of losing is disavowed in mainstream and naive approaches to the phenomenon, which tend to overlook how aggressivity is constitutive of subjectivity.

The last crossroads is the role identification and imago play in the 'free market' economy and the most essential goods sold there: ourselves, whether buying identities to 'express who we are' or being bought by labor psychology that tells us 'who we are.' The mirror stage offers important lessons on how the imago and the concept of identity are captured in today's neoliberal market, which provides the illusion of celebrating the self only under the condition of being able to instrumentalize and exploit that same celebration.

These intersections proposed by Lacan offer a new way to approach a key psychoanalytic lesson in a contemporary environment: subjectivity is not simply a product of socio-historical influences, nor is there an authentic kernel of spontaneous subjectivity, but a tension along the lines of our symbolic life and image of ourselves, a tension in our 'animal' nature, a tension in our 'violent' relations towards others, a tension in our 'identity.'

A final chapter will discuss how the Lacanian mirror stage enables us to go beyond the Imaginary traps provoked by today's media and cultural landscape, using the aphorism mentioned at the end of the mirror stage text, *Thou art that* (*You are that*), and in the brief analysis of a recent film that deals with something monstruous the subject cannot control within itself.

One last point: perhaps, it could be useful to have a few lines on the use of a concept as complex as *identity* in the framework of cultural studies, a body of works and authors that, it seems to me, is the one that has most intensely reflected on such question as something central to its theoretical work.[3] Stuart Hall (1996, pp. 1–2) says that the theoretical problem of this much-discussed concept lies in locating how to work through such concepts, or else to locate in what precise ways their use is irreducible: in other words, with concepts as complex as *identity*, we must pass the inertia of saying, once again, what others have already said, and, rather, go through that discussion while delimiting the conditions of what is minimally necessary to sustain the existence of the concept. In the same text, Hall reflects on the advantages and disadvantages of the key places of the debate on identity in which the problem was founded for cultural studies: mainly in Althusser, Lacan,

Foucault and Butler. Hall provides a good introduction to the Lacanian approach to the concept, for the function of the Other in the constitution of identity is recognized, as well as its impossibility of completion. However, as we shall see, these ideas are not sufficient to grasp Lacan's point, for what Hall fails to grasp is that it is not a matter of a "binary" (p. 9) logic of the constitution of the subject, but of a paradox in that constitution: as will be explained in more detail in the rest of the work, the matter is not reduced to a linear logic in which, first, one *is not* a subject, *then* comes the mirror stage, and one *is now* a subject; rather, the subject inhabits a paradox of causality in its constitution through the Other. This, among many other things, is what cultural studies do not seem to grasp when criticizing psychoanalysis as 'binary,' for they assume that when psychoanalysis exhibits a 'binary logic,' it is because it recognizes the two 'parts' of that binarism as already constituted beforehand, two halves that make a complete unit or that one part is privileged over the other.[4]

Now, let's start with Freud.

Notes

1 The chaotic (to say the least) variety of translations and versions of Lacan's Seminar is something to be worked through on another project (as it has been in many before). I am not blind to objections (as some I have raised myself in some places) on using the *millerian* version (published in French by De Seuil and in English by W.W. Norton & Company and Polity): it is indisputable that those are the most widely circulated and popular versions; whether those are 'the best versions' is something to be discussed elsewhere. On the other hand, I will be using the 'updated' version of the whole compilation of *écrits* in English (Bruce Finks' 2006 translation), but it might be useful to remember that even though those texts were compiled in 1966, they were previously published in many places before (thus the years in parenthesis); in addition, it could be important to remember those years to situate ourselves chronologically, for Lacan made several modifications when the texts became part of the compilation in 1966. Ángel de Frutos Salvador (1994) has made, to my knowledge, the best work in comparing each version of each *écrit*. On my part, I will mention the year of the *écrit* when introducing it, but I will always quote the year as 1966 for I am working with the compilation.

2 In the case of Freud, I will be using the 'previous' Standard Edition. Even though the advantages of the most recent collection, the one supervised by Mark Solms, I presume the 'original' Strachey edition is still much more popular today. Thus, I will add in parenthesis the year of the edition of the volume I am quoting, and the Roman numeral of that volume.

3 It is not my intention to put this text within the framework of cultural studies (it is a text on Lacanian psychoanalysis), but, as I have experienced, there seems to be some inertia that compels us to write about how a concept has been used in other fields. This creates a sort of 'proof' that we are being interdisciplinary, but that is questionable: just because we quote again an author or body of works doesn't mean we engage with them or that we are actually working in an interdisciplinary fashion.

4 The key place to dispel this misunderstanding is Joan Copjec's book (1994), especially the last chapter.

References

Copjec, Jean. [1994] (2015). *Read My Desire: Lacan Against the Historicists.* Verso.

Freud, Sigmund. [1911–1915] (1958). "Papers on Technique." In *The Standard Edition of The Complete Psychological Works of Sigmund Freud*, Vol. XII. The Hogarth Press, pp. 83–173.

Freud, Sigmund. [1921] (1955). "Group Psychology and the Analysis of the Ego." In *The Standard Edition of The Complete Psychological Works of Sigmund Freud*, Vol. XVIII. The Hogarth Press, pp. 65–143.

Hall, Stuart. (1996). "Introduction: Who Needs Identity?" In Stuart Hall & Paul du Gay (eds.), *Questions of Cultural Identity.* Sage Publications, pp. 1–17.

Lacan, Jacques. [1949] (2006). "The Mirror Stage as Formative of the *I* Function as Revealed in Psychoanalytic Experience." In *Écrits. The First Complete Edition in English.* W.W. Norton & Company, pp. 75–81.

Reiss, Diana & Marino, Lori. (2001). "Mirror self-recognition in the bottlenose dolphin: A case of cognitive convergence." *Proceedings of the National Academy of Sciences of the United States of America*, Vol. 98, No. 10, pp. 5937–5942.

Salvador, Ángel de Frutos. (1994). *Los Escritos de Jacques Lacan. Variantes textuales.* Siglo XXI.

2

FREUDIAN IDENTIFICATION

Two Paths

Within the work of Freud, we can discern two important paths that lead us to the concept of identification: first, the one opened by transference, especially the one sustained in the relationship between analyst and analysand; second, the one opened in masses, where identification is understood as a mental infection.

On transference as identification

One of the most important pivot points in the theoretical development of psychoanalysis is the discovery of what Freud called *transference*, and more precisely, the discovery of how psychoanalysis can operate with transference.

The first Freudian text devoted exclusively to this topic was presented in the "Papers on technique" series, was published in 1912 and is entitled *The Dynamics of Transference* (Freud, 1958/XII). It is short in length, but particularly incisive in Freud's thought, since the protagonist is a concept that, although it can be traced as back as 1895 in *Studies on Hysteria* (Freud and Breuer, 1955/II), and even occupies a famous postscript to the Dora case in 1905 (Freud, 1953/VII), had not been explicitly worked on by its author in any theoretical writing.

Freud begins *The Dynamics of Transference* by admitting how normal it is in human life that, due to the impressions and influences received during childhood (and *especially* in childhood), the subject

> has acquired a specific method of his own in his conduct of his erotic life—that is, in the preconditions to falling in love which he lays down, in the instincts he satisfies and the aims he sets himself in the course of it.
>
> *(1958/XII, p. 99)*

DOI: 10.4324/9781003640653-2

In other words, each person is uniquely determined to behave in his erotic (not only sexual) relationships in a way that stages the influences he received from erotic relationships during his childhood, so that one can verify a certain pattern of erotic/love dynamics that appear in a subject's life from the pattern of love dynamics the subject had when going through childhood. These love relationships are not to be understood only in the romantic and/or sexual sense, but in a broader sense that would include friendships, those whom we admire and respect, and even those whom we dislike.

What today seems to be popular wisdom, because it is, perhaps, so obvious to us, is something Freud indicates should be also applied to the relations analysands have with their analysts, so that it will be inevitable to "introduce the [analyst] into one of the psychical 'series' which the patient has already formed" (p. 100), it is a revivification of "the subject's infantile imagos" (p. 102). Already here, the Lacanian word appears.

Freud recognizes that, in its early beginnings, psychoanalysis did not take transference seriously, and operated with *suggestion*, the latter being "the influencing of a person by means of the transference phenomena which are possible in his case" (p. 106). Thus, suggestion works on a transference *already* installed: one can be suggested because one has *already* established a transference relationship with the suggester, so that one allows oneself to be influenced in action, thought and/or feeling.

What, then, would be the difference between suggestion and transference? Psychoanalytic transference is not so much the influence that the analyst has on his analysand, or the subordination that the analysand assumes towards his analyst, but the *dynamics* in which the analysand repeats, in his relationship with his analyst, that staging of the conditions of his love life. And unlike the many other spaces where we work with suggestion, the two fundamental rules of psychoanalysis, free association and evenly suspended attention,[1] make possible a device that is not governed by the meaning of the utterances as the daily dialogue we have on everyday life. *Transference is constructed* in the analytic device itself.

As the analysis progresses and penetrates into certain complexes of the analysand's relations with others and the dynamics of symptomatic formation, coincidences begin to emerge between those same complexes and dynamics with the analytic work itself; that is, in the analytic device, the transferential relations that the analysand sustains outside the device seem to be staged within the analytical work, so that the analyst is inserted in this series of relations, and it is this insertion that occupies an extremely fundamental work in the analysis. It would not be an exaggeration to think that one comes to analysis suffering from something, and the first thing that analysis gives in return, and in which its functioning is verified, is that one seems to worsen or repeat what one already suffers from in one's relationships with the analyst.

Let us not fall into the naivety, Freud warns us (p. 105), of believing that when the analysand has a 'good' relationship with his analyst, then we are dealing with a 'good' transference, as if that is the only transference that works. Whether there are feelings of very high esteem and admiration, or aggressiveness and hostility, the point is to manage to locate those feelings towards the analyst as a staging of a certain repetition of the relations the analysand has towards others. The contingent features of the analyst, its[2] sex and name especially, exercise a certain influence too in this staging (and in particular cases, even such things as where the consultation is located, or the color of the couch).

In short, this first Freudian conception of identification is the recognition of transference as *the staging of a certain type of repetition*: in the relationship that the analysand sustains towards its analyst, a certain dynamic of the singular symptomatic formations of the subject is verified, as well as the way in which the subject has sustained relationships with others in the past. Analysis is not simply constructed as a space where the analysand speaks and the analyst listens and interprets, but one where *the relationship between analyst and analysand* is inserted as the condition for that which is spoken and listened to and interpreted: analysis ceases to be a place where one communicates something to the other, and begins to be a place where one communicates *in relation to the other.*

On identification as infection

The second path of Freudian identification is the one extensively worked on in 1921's *Group Psychology and the Analysis of the Ego* (Freud, 1955/XVIII). In that work, identification is defined as "the earliest expression of an emotional tie with another person" (p. 105), something that "endeavours to mould a person's own ego after the fashion of the one that has been taken as a model" (p. 106). This *configuration of one's ego in fashion of another as a model* does not refer only to a process in which the ego aspires to be *like* another person—for example, as when we try to imitate those things that the other does, or try to follow the advice that the other gives us. Even in these moments, it is difficult to establish why I am really interested in doing what the other does, or why I am really interested in following the advice.

The identifications that psychoanalysis is most interested in are those that function unconsciously, beyond the realm of the ego, like an unconscious identification with a behavior, an object, a position or a situation. An obvious example of a behavioral identification is the infectious capacity of accents: when we travel to a different region where there is an accent different from ours, it is common that we begin to copy it, even without intending to or noticing it, unless someone lets us know. Another very common example is how we repeat the phrases, gestures or even ways of using our body of those with whom we spend more time, such as our partner or friends. It seems, in these cases, that we cannot avoid copying the other, identifying ourselves with the other.

Freud located in the mechanism of identification a *symptom* that, as such, revealed *a certain arrangement of subjectivity*. Freud reminds us of the case of Dora text (1955/XVIII, pp. 106–107), who had a cough through identification with the also coughing father, in order to occupy the place that the father had in the amorous plot of the K couple: via a behavior such as coughing, Dora unconsciously identified herself with her father in order to occupy his place and consummate, as Freud read *a posteriori* in the case published (1953/VII), a homosexual fantasy with Mrs. K.

Identification thus functions so that the subject obtains pleasure or avoids displeasure. In the case of an identification with objects, we can only look around an inhabited space to realize how the objects that attract or repel us represent an identifying bridge with an ideal or with the psychical series Freud talks about. How common it is to notice an unconscious externalization of a friend just by looking at the places he frequents, the clothes he wears, the pets he has, the music he listens to or the books he reads: it is the identification through an object that condenses a certain nucleus of our own subjectivity.

In the case of positions, we verify the identification by putting ourselves, unconsciously, 'in the other's shoes.' This is the case of the analysand who, when speaking of his sister, makes mistakes by referring to her in the first person (as if *he is* the sister); or the analysand who, when speaking of her friend's partner, speaks of her friend in the first person (as if her friend's partner is *her own*). These identifications are symptomatic because they reveal a certain unconscious subjective arrangement: via these lapsus that point to a positional identification, a certain unconscious resentment between siblings is revealed, or a certain infatuation with the friend's partner.

In the case of situations, we also come across them frequently in our own relationships or in those of others. This is the case of the typical man who complains that 'women are all the same': could it be that they are all the same, or that he always repeats the same situation in his relationship with women? It is the case of the woman who complains that she 'always ends up with louts': to what extent is she responsible for finding herself in the same situation, over and over again, when relating to men?

These identifications end up in what Freud describes as "mental infection," in which identification occurs "based upon the possibility or desire of putting oneself in the same situation [as the other's]" (p. 107). This is the case when I see someone suffering, say, from the death of her mother, and I begin to feel sadness because I imagine how I would feel if my mother died, or I remember when my mother died. Freud warns (p. 107) that we should not confuse this with sympathy, because for sympathy to occur, one must *already* have identified oneself: for some reason, we feel more that kind of sadness when the other is a close friend than when it is a stranger.

Thus, Freud placed identification as a process even more primordial than sympathy for the other, or even before any interest for the other. In the film

Midsommar (dir. Ari Aster, 2019), in a scene near the climax, the protagonist begins to cry out loud in desperation, and the women around her start to imitate her cries: far from this being out of sympathy (since those women are part of the community that kidnapped her group), it is via showing themselves identified with her that they make her part of the community.[3]

Lacan managed to locate more precisely this precedence of unconscious identification over any conscious, moral empathy or sympathy for the other. He did it by locating identification at the very heart of the birth of subjectivity, that the very idea of the Self only arises through the other.

Notes

1 For a comment on these rules, especially the second, see another paper on technique: 1912's *Recommendations to Physicians Practicing Psychoanalysis* (1958/XII).

2 I use the pronoun 'it' to emphasize the impersonal and objectual feature of the analyst and the analysand.

3 This scene seems to be an adaptation of a story that Freud relates in the first part of *The Interpretation of Dreams* (Freud, 1958/IV): after a doctor reviewed the symptoms of a hysterical attack, the other patients there also began to have it. Referring to this example, Freud indicates that "identification is not simple imitation but assimilation on the basis of a similar aetiological pretension" (p. 150); that is, to identify oneself is not simply to imitate, but to introject, to make one's own, to become involved in what the other does.

References

Freud, Sigmund. [1900] (1958). "The Interpretation of Dreams (First Part)." In *The Standard Edition of The Complete Psychological Works of Sigmund Freud*, Vol. IV. The Hogarth Press.

Freud, Sigmund. [1905] (1953). "Fragment of an Analysis of a Case of Hysteria." In *The Standard Edition of The Complete Psychological Works of Sigmund Freud*, Vol. VII. The Hogarth Press, pp. 2–122.

Freud, Sigmund. [1912] (1958). "The Dynamics of Transference." In *The Standard Edition of The Complete Psychological Works of Sigmund Freud*, Vol. XII. The Hogarth Press, pp. 97–108.

Freud, Sigmund. [1912] (1958). "Recommendations to Physicians Practicing Psychoanalysis." In *The Standard Edition of The Complete Psychological Works of Sigmund Freud*, Vol. XII. The Hogarth Press, pp. 109–120.

Freud, Sigmund. [1921] (1955). "Group Psychology and the Analysis of the Ego." In *The Standard Edition of The Complete Psychological Works of Sigmund Freud*, Vol. XVIII. The Hogarth Press, pp. 65–143.

Freud, Sigmund & Breuer, Josef. [1895] (1955). "Studies on Hysteria." In *The Standard Edition of The Complete Psychological Works of Sigmund Freud*, Vol. II. The Hogarth Press.

3

LACANIAN IDENTIFICATION

An Imago for the Subject

The ego, the other and reality in Freud's *Project*

Before entering *The Mirror Stage*, we should do one more stop. In 1895, inspired by his recent collaboration with Joseph Breuer, Freud began to draft a document never published during his lifetime, which was discovered posthumously and which we know today as *Project for a Scientific Psychology* (Freud, 1966/I; in what follows, *Project*). This text constitutes a kind of hinge where the last glimpses of Freud's neurological interest can be seen, but already subordinated to his growing interest in understanding the human psyche.

One of the most interesting points of the *Project* is that Freud poses the relation of the subject to the world around him in terms of pleasure and displeasure. Displeasure is an elevation of tension on the perceiving system, while pleasure is the discharge of this tension, so that pleasure and displeasure are the "intercommunicating vessels" between the perceiving system and the psychic system (p. 312); that is, the relation between what our senses capture from the world and the psychic system that processes it is regulated by a logic of displeasure (excitation) and pleasure (discharge). The relationship established between these communicating vessels has the function of constituting the ego (*Ich*).

Two crucial points arise here. The first is that this relation of pleasure–displeasure is not only sustained with one's own body, but also with one's *fellow human-being* (*Nebenmensch*), with another person:

> Let us suppose that the object which furnishes the perception resembles the subject—a *fellow human-being*. If so, the theoretical interest [taken in it] is also explained by the fact that an object *like this* was simultaneously

DOI: 10.4324/9781003640653-3

> the [subject's] first satisfying object and further his first hostile object, as well as his sole helping power. For this reason it is in relation to a fellow human-being that a human-being learns to cognize.
>
> *(Freud, 1966/I, p. 331)*

It turns out, then, that one finds in the other (in the other person, the fellow human-being) a possibility of feeling pleasure *and* displeasure: the relationship with the other brings this ambivalence, it is at the same time something foreign and something internal, it is an object of the external world and, at the same time, it leads back to "memories of quite similar visual impressions of his own" (p. 331)—that is, of ego's own body. Freud has just realized, via the pleasure–displeasure relation, *how fundamental the other is for the constitution of the ego*: the ego is constituted through *cognizing* the other, to discern the other from the self, a matter that, later in his work, Freud understood as *identification*.

The second crucial point is that, through this pleasure–displeasure system, the ego manages to create a relation of *communication* (p. 366) between itself and the world: among the perceptions of the world, there are those pleasant and those unpleasant, and in the unpleasant group, Freud indicates (p. 366), bodily enervations (screaming, crying, pain in the body) are also knotted. The unpleasurable does not presuppose an intrinsic quality in the object, but is found in the *association* that this object has with bodily enervation, an association that is sustained in conscious memory; that is, the function that memory has for the human organism is to prevent the ego from coming into contact with that object that provokes an enervation of pain: "the *information of one's own [reaction]* serves to characterize the object" (p. 366). So far, it seems that the only lesson from this is that memory has a survival function.

But let us see the conclusion drawn from all this: "Not much is now needed in order to invent speech. There are other objects, which constantly produce certain sounds—in whose perceptual complex, that is, a sound plays a part" (p. 367). We see here that Freud *derives the creation of speech as the result of the association of the external object with the body*: speech and language is a product of the pleasure–displeasure system—that is to say, a product of the relation of the ego with the world.

We find in the *Project* two elements that will be key in the articulation that will come in the next chapters: (1) the other and the self are not constituted as two isolated spheres, but *one in relation to the other*, in an intersubjective relation (to say it in Lacanian), and (2) language is a structure that conditions the relation that the self has with the external world, so that *language* and *understanding of the world* are not two independent issues; thus, the problem in understanding the world *is* a problem of language that language itself *cannot* solve.

In short: when the ego initiates a relationship with the external world, this relationship is always already mediated as a crossroads with the other, and it is in the symbolic function of language that the impossibility for the ego to build a transparent and direct relationship with the other and with the world becomes evident.

Let's get into the Lacanian text on the mirror stage, which will be complemented with some ideas from *Presentation on Psychical Causality* and *Beyond the "Reality Principle"*.

The birth of the ego in Lacan's *Mirror*

A few paragraphs into *The Mirror Stage*, a definition of the concept of its title is given through identification and imago:

> It suffices to understand the mirror stage in this context *as an identification*, in the full sense analysis gives to the term: namely, the transformation that takes place in the subject when he assumes *[assume]* an image—an image that is seemingly predestined to have an effect at this phase, as witnessed by the use in analytic theory of antiquity's term, "imago."
>
> *(Lacan, 1966, p. 76)*

In order to understand the consequences of the subject assuming an image, let us take this formulation as a compass in the argument: *identification is the process by which the ego assumes an image as its own identity, so that it receives its own identity from the other.*

What is new in *The Mirror Stage* is that the idea of the *imago* that Freud barely sketched or supposed, in Lacan acquires a preponderant and very definite function.

At this point, it is important to have a little digression in a translation issue (and the advantages it could bring). When we read in an English Lacan the word "ego," most of the time it translates the French "moi," which refers to the Freudian "Ich" (take, as an example, the title of the first Seminar). Sometimes, people refer to *ego* and *I* as synonymous, a decision that I don't necessarily disagree with. However, in English, there is another word that comes to mind when dealing with these concepts, self, which has caused a little discussion within psychoanalytic community. It is not in my interest to be part of such debate, for I take it as a translation issue, so, what is the difference, for the purposes of this work, between *ego* and *self*? I propose the following: let's take Lacan's definition, mentioned above, and use imago as a synonym of self. The self is an image, *found in the outside reality*, into which the subject identifies *itself*: there's the proper pun, *the subject finds it(s)self outside.* The ego, on the other hand, is the psychic process of identification "that takes place in the subject when he assumes *[assume]* an image."

Thus, ego is found within, self is found outside. Following this logic, the previous chapter on Freudian identification could be rewritten as an identification towards objects, situations, images and/or others of *my/self*. This way to distinguish ego and self explains why, as we will see in the following chapters, zoologists talk about *the animal ego* (for they talk about cognitive process in the animals), the selfie is, as its name implies, an *object/self of my ego*, identity politics are preoccupied with images of the self, and labor psychology 'studies' the ego in order to produce an identification with a self.[1] In addition, as might already be noticed, I intend to use *subject* with the pronoun *it*, instead of using both masculine and feminine pronouns, for the Lacanian subject is not defined as a gendered individual, and, on some occasions, I might use *her/him* precisely to talk about the psychological individual (or the ego), not the Lacanian subject. Now, back to the text.

The imago is the result, in the ego, of *having assumed as its own an image given from the exteriority*: when the ego assumes an image, which we call *self*, it is transformed; a cut is produced in it, leaving a state prior and a state subsequent to identification. The mirror stage is the moment of this first transformation, which then constitutes the birth of the subject itself: prior to this first identification, there is no subject, since there is no transformation of, but a *constitution towards*. That is to say, the first transformation, given in the infant who assumes an image as his own, is not the passage from 'subject X' to 'subject Y', but the creation of a subject where before there was nothing more than a biological organism. We distinguish, then, the biological organism (whose functioning is explained to us by anatomy) from the subject that is assumed as the one that inhabits that organism.

Up to this point, it would seem that we are in developmental psychology, as if these were natural phases already predisposed in the human body that have no relation with otherness, so that the mirror stage would be a *natural* pivot point between two differentiated states. What happens then? The human infant has a moment, between six and 18 months of age, where he seems to recognize his own image in the mirror—that is, where he recognizes that *what appears elsewhere*, in the mirror, *is it(s)self*. The infant has a "jubilant assumption" (p. 76) of his image.[2]

There are several elements that participate in this identificatory process: the other, which is what *offers* the subject an image, and the subject, who is constituted as such by *assuming* that image. The subject identifies his own self with what the other offers him, so that any attempt by the subject to formulate his own identity can only be done by going through the other.

The infant recognizes in an image *that is given to him from outside*, that which he *is*. This first image is an imaginary self, "the ideal-I" (p. 76). It is the self that corresponds to what our senses capture, it is the self that functions through a correspondence between the body and the interiority, it is the self that responds to self-consciousness. *The primary function of the mirror stage is to offer a union, called* imago, *between the body and the self.*

A defective joint

But there is a catch here. This exteriority, Lacan warns us (p. 76), "is more constitutive than constituted": there is a price the ego pays for constituting itself through the image. When the subject assumes that image as its own, the subject does not simply see itself as *already* constituted in it, it does not simply verify, through the image, what it *already* is; in turn, the subject is constituted *in* the image. *Constitution of the subject*, in Lacanian, is then read in these two ways: as something that *constitutes the subject* and as something in which *the subject is constituted.* These two ways appear synchronically: the subject is not already constituted and then verified in the image, nor does the image alone constitute the subject as if the subject were a passive block of clay. That is why the other has a preponderant function: *the other gives the subject an image that the subject assumes.*

Let us see how he explains it in a text from 1936. In *Beyond the "Reality Principle"*, Lacan tells us that the Freudian imago has an "*informational* function in intuition, memory and development" (p. 71). That function, which informs because it *gives form*, is at the heart of the process of identification, which Lacan separates from imitation:

> [*Identification*] is quite different from the process of *imitation*, which is distinguished by its partial and groping form of approximation; *identification* contrasts with imitation not simply as the *global* assimilation of a structure but as the *virtual assimilation of development* implied by that structure in a still undifferentiated state.
>
> *(p. 71)*

Identification with the *imago* is identification with a structure at a given moment that has subsequent developmental effects. As we shall see later, this is what made him so interested in the development of animals.

Let's return to *The Mirror Stage.* Whereas identity could be understood as something that the subject 'appropriates,' 'resignifies' or 'constructs' (which are ways in which racial, sexual, gender, political or ideological identity struggles are often explained)—that is, whereas identity is understood as something that *emanates from* the subject, or that the subject *has*—for psychoanalysis, identification is a process of constitution *from the other*, so there is no identity in itself, but a continuous process of identifications that provides a place of alienation for the subject.

Then, *the subject is the result of an alienation in his identifications, not the agent of his own identity.* [3] Identity here is not seen as a place of freedom for the subject, but as a deception in which the subject attempts to condense and tame the process of unconscious identifications.

Thus, the subject *is constituted* in the imago, which has the *function of offering a kind of union*: between the interiority of the body and the exterior image of this body. While the image is the sum of visible characteristics that are reflected in the mirror, or the sum of quantitative data that describe what we are or do, the *imago* is the result of *assuming* that those characteristics and those data *are myself*: the imago arises because there is a taking of position with respect to what one assumes that one is or is not. While the image is simply exteriority (say, what the mirror reflects), the imago is the resulting effect of that union between the image and the interiority of the body (the way in which the subject is involved with that which the mirror reflects).

For Lacan, the imago is so powerful for the constitution of the subject that it uses the image (what the mirror reflects) as the "threshold of the visible world" (p. 77), as something that has the primary function of "establishing a relationship between an organism and its reality" (p. 78). In other words, the ego relates to the objects of reality through the imago already assumed by it. The imago is the subject's passport to the world of reality: thanks to the function of the imago as a glue, the subject *obtains* a body that offers it a certain support for relating to others.

What Freud called "psychical series," those in which the subject identified the others with whom it relates, Lacan called "*ideal identifications*" (p. 145), which form a trajectory that accounts for the function of the imago in the subject. These ideal identifications are organized into something we know as the *ego*: the ego is, then, the series of repetitions of ideal identifications upon which subjectivity is constituted. In this way, Lacan tries to move away from any conception of subjectivity that attempts "a subjective synthesis [defined in] objective terms" (p. 145)[4]—that is, a conception of subjectivity that tries to account for singularity from a closure/synthesis, and does not understand it as a continuous opening.

But there is something this imago, this glue, cannot keep together. The imago breaks apart the subject and the ego:

> But the important point is that [the ideal-I] situates the agency known as the ego [*moi*], prior to its social determination, in a fictional direction that will forever remain irreducible for any single individual or, rather, that will only asymptotically approach the subject's becoming, no matter how successful the dialectical syntheses by which he must resolve, as *I* [*je*], his discordance with his own reality.
>
> *(Lacan, 1966, p. 76)*

How to understand this idea? This is where the distinction given between *moi* and *je* becomes important, which is why I put them in brackets in the quotation. While there is an ego/I (*moi*) that presents itself in our conscious acts, and that is the ego/I of which I speak when I speak of myself, there is another I (*je*) that exists only *as a function*, or let us say, it exists as a kind of orthopedics that allows the conscious I to function, and it is the I that does not correspond to the self, an *I* that dwells outside the I of the image. One is the I of the individual, the other is the I of the subject.

The subject is what hinders the complete construction of the ego in the individual. We could here place the formula that *the individual is at a disjoint towards its own completeness because of the subject.*

If, as Lacan told us a little while ago, the mirror stage is the moment of the first "transformation that takes place in the subject when he assumes an image," and if we can call this transformation an *identification*, then we find the price paid for obtaining this identification: *the existence of the subject as a function*, which causes the I to live a perpetual "discordance with his own reality." The subject is the result of the effort of the imago trying to secure the union between the I of the image and the body that is assumed in that image.

This subject is one that has a function "irreducible for any single individual": the subject, subject of enunciation, subject of language, will never correspond to the individual who speaks, the I of the utterances, the I of the image. The subject is something *excessive* to the individual who speaks, and at the same time *is less* than the individual who speaks. Far from this constituting a 'deformation' or a 'problem' of the ego, it is constitutive of itself: for psychoanalysis, the ego inhabits a constitutive split that prevents it from acquiring its own completeness, that forces it to be always alienated from itself.

The body and its organs

Why can't we have a causal, direct correspondence between the ego and the body? Why does the body behave as an otherness for the ego? One of the key lessons of psychoanalysis is that the body seems to enjoy (by) itself, partially, as if the body organs run amok in enjoyment. This is the way in which otherness of its own body presents to the ego: as if the body is always fragmented.

When we point out that the body enjoys itself in a fragmented way, we are referring to a key issue introduced by Freud in the second of his *Three Essays on Sexuality.* These are the *erotogenic zones*, defined as "a part of the skin or mucous membrane in which stimuli which produce the pleasure are governed by special conditions" (Freud, 1953/VII, p. 183). In other words, the erotogenic zones are a part of the body (most frequently an orifice such as the mouth, the anus, the urethra, the nose, the eyes, the ears) which, because of their biological functioning in constant stimulation, are charged with a specific pleasure that functions beyond biological need: this is how one explains that children suck their thumb, which does not satisfy their hunger, due to the pleasure that, having been linked to the pleasure of satisfying hunger, sucking produces in the mouth.

To understand this, let us stay with the most obvious example, and the first one Freud deals with. The baby cries because of hunger, and cannot, unlike other animals, satisfy this need without help from the other.[5] The mother gives the infant milk, which the infant sucks with one of the orifices of its body, the mouth, and thus succeeds in satisfying a *biological need* for survival. In turn, then, there is an object in the world, the mother's breast, which is *the object of the satisfaction* of this biological need. If need demands X, and satisfaction delivers X, thus resulting in a homeostatic state, we can summarize this process in the formula $N - S = 0$ (Need – Satisfaction = Homeostasis).

Now, as Freud conjectured in the *Project* (1966/I, p. 319), that satisfaction, when *remembered*, produces a kind of *state of split perception* (my words, not Freud's): I have the memory of that experience of satisfaction, but I am not being satisfied in reality. The mouth, that part of the body with which the satisfaction had been experienced, has been charged with a certain erotogenic quality; it is libidinized, it has been invested with a certain veil of satisfaction that *exceeds* the biological need for which it exists: because of memories, I feel pleasure, but this pleasure, which is not one that corresponds to reality (I can distinguish this pleasure in memory from the actual pleasure in reality), produces a *desire* that exceeds its biological satisfaction. By giving me the breast to feed me through the mouth and calm my hunger, the other not only satisfies my biological need but also gives me *something additional*: the other also satisfies the excitement produced by the memory of that satisfaction. There is, then, in satisfying my need, something *extra* that is given by the satisfaction of the need itself: the human does not live in that homeostatic state where the satisfaction of the need is simply subtracted from the need, but there remains a kind of *residue*, which is the satisfaction of satisfying the need. The formula would be $N - S + S^S = D$ (Need – Satisfaction + Satisfaction of Satisfaction = Desire).[6]

Thus, erotogenic zones are evidence of how the body seems to seek and achieve certain satisfaction outside the will of the ego, and although certain logics of the biological functioning of the human body make some parts especially erotogenized (the mouth for the need to feed, the anus for the need to defecate, the urethra for the need to urinate), the dynamics of erotogenization of these or any other part is very singular in each person. An analysand, in her first sessions, gives an account of the things with which she feels dissatisfied in life, especially in the sexual and friendship spheres. At one point, while telling an anecdote, she says that "fue la gota que derramó el *brazo*… perdón, el *vaso*."[7] She is then asked to talk about the *brazo* (arm), not so much the *vaso* (glass), and very soon she indicates that since she was a child, she felt great satisfaction and pride in her own arms, shaped by her physical activity and with particularly well-cared-for skin… with her lapsus, the arm appeared, trying to take the floor. It is a body that speaks at the margin of the I, as if within the I there were a division that constantly splits it in two: between the I and the other.

My body (?)

It is in language, as in the confusion between the glass and the arm, where we notice that split in which the ego constantly dwells and which does not allow it to be in harmony even with its own body. Let's see some examples of this.

This is something we experience every day in our daily speech. We arrive at a house, we ring the bell at the entrance and from the intercom someone asks, "Who is here?" and we answer, "It's me": don't we notice here a splitting of the "I" in *It* is *me*? Do we take our self as an it?

Language is that which not only allows but *forces* the "I" to be something else. When we are asked how to get to a certain place, it is common for us to *position our body* as if we were in front of a street or building, to use our hands to indicate the turns and even to pretend that we are the other person, in order to give a precise indication of where to look. The saying 'putting yourself in someone else's shoes' takes a quite literal meaning: the human being is the one who constantly seems to want to *usurp* the other person's body. The realization of how we use our own body as a puppet is what allows psychoanalysis to move away from a psychologization for which all thought is inside the individual: we may think with the brain, but in everyday life we very often think with the rest of the body, and even with the body of others.

This allows Lacan to call human space a *kaleidoscopic geometry* (p. 99): just as the image in a kaleidoscope creates new patterns as it moves, so the subject can project its own subjectivity in different ways, but always in the field of the other: *subjectivity is condemned to traverse the field of the other*. I am condemned to always conceive myself as an(other).[8]

This idea of conceiving oneself as an(other) is at the very heart of subjectivity, specifically, in the relationship that the "I" maintains with its own body. It is quite shocking for some people to learn that the image we see of ourselves in the mirror is not the way we are seen by others, due to the optical effect of inversion of the mirror itself: once, in a photography class, I noticed the enormous surprise, even loaded with displeasure, when, with digital tools, a photo of a person was flipped and a somewhat uncanny image appeared, a version of us that we recognize as such but that is strange to us at the same time. It also happens outside the visual realm because, as the imago is constructed with the senses, we obtain a phenomenon similar to that of the inverted photo when we listen for the first time to a recording of our voice: suddenly, it seems that the body we have is not really ours, that the voice is not ours. The same thing happens when we see a caricature of us, or someone imitates us: it seems that there is something in our physical appearance, our speaking or behavior that, while representing us for the other, is *excessive* (just like the features that are exaggerated in a caricature or a parodic imitation): it is something ours, but it seems that it is *too much* ours; it seems that we do not even *completely* control the body we have, as if something in it escapes our power.

This is precisely the split Lacan speaks of about the human subject having a body, and it must be understood in this way: it *has* a body, but its body does not correspond to the I that inhabits it; rather, there is a fundamental split between the I and the body—that is to say, the I has a body, but it is not easy to say that its body *belongs* to it.

This psychoanalytic understanding goes directly against the psychologizing discourses that pretend to make the "I" correspond to its body, as we can attest in those moments when psychologists ask the patient to look in the mirror and say something out loud *to himself*, or to write a message to be read every day in front of the mirror ('Accept yourself,' 'Have courage,' 'A new me' are the ones I have heard).

What we encounter in this sort of generic formulas that discourses such as psychological *coaching* propagate is the representation of a definition of *psychologization: the attempt to establish a correspondence between the ego and its body*; that is to say, psychologization is the attempt to make the imago consist, to pretend that the imago establishes (not a disjoint, but) a direct and authentic correspondence between the ego and the body. Psychoanalysis operates, precisely, *against* the imago; it operates on the assumption that the imago is deceptive, that it "alienates [the human] from himself" (p. 92).

Psychoanalysis is skeptical of contemporary syntagms such as 'mental health,' and various other 'syndromes' that characterize human subjectivity today, and despite the fact that we so often hear how openly people say they have this or that 'mental problem' or 'mental illness' (from 'anxiety syndrome' to 'depression,' 'ADHD' and 'autism spectrum'), it is not unusual to find that this very precise diagnosis has no effect whatsoever on subjectivity: it is as if by having a precise etiquette for its 'disease,' the subject can *reinforce* the attitudes, behaviors and relationships with others that define, precisely, the disease. It is common to hear analysands in their first sessions saying that *because of* the abuse or violence they suffered in childhood, or very specific family problems, they *know* that this is *why* they have problems with substance abuse, in their relationships with food or violent behavior with others, and *yet*, despite being able to locate the specific reasons for this, they don't understand why they can't change. It is as if the psychological *knowledge* has no effect on subjectivity: 'I know, and yet I continue as if I don't know' is a commonplace in our world so hyperdiagnosed by today's psychology.

The psychology that seeks to strengthen the "I" is committed to making the subject correspond to his body, to offer the "I" a very precise account of what it suffers, of what its body suffers, but don't human condition and experience demonstrate exactly the opposite, that it is very difficult to give a precise account of our own suffering?

So common is this experience of estrangement within one's own body that it is the subject of memes: three persons violently kicking on the floor another one who begs them to stop; all of them have written "me." And we can find a fourth "me": the I that assumes such a cartoon as a moment in its life. The *I* operates, sometimes, outside of the self, and even seems to operate *against the self.* [9] Another meme I once read expressed this excessiveness of the subject that cannot be comprised even within the individual: "Richard Ashcroft [the vocalist of rock band The Verve] can be as much Richard Ashcroft as he wants, but he will never know what it feels like to walk down the street feeling like Richard Ashcroft in the *Bitter Sweet Symphony* video."

When I was a kid, I was playing hide-and-seek with my cousin and sister at my grandmother's big old house. At one point, when I was seeking, I 'saw' my cousin at the end of a big hall and I screamed at him, "I've seen you!" I repeated it many times, and since he didn't come out of his hiding spot, I said he was cheating. It was only after I took a few steps towards him that I realized I was screaming at my own reflection in the mirror at the end of the hall. It was through the misrecognition of my own figure that I thought I had caught the other.[10]

The mirror stage allows Lacan (p. 79) to characterize human subjectivity, in "socially elaborated situations," via three main consequences vectors: (1) it is mediated *by the desire of the other*, (2) it mutates *rivalry with the other* into objects, and (3) it *places the subject in a position alienated* from any natural process. In other words, the great conclusion of the mirror stage is that this split between the ego and the body from which the subject is born shows us that human subjectivity cannot not pass through the other, it manages to tame an aggressiveness towards the other by directing it now towards objects, and it places us, because of the existence of the subject, in a place that does not correspond only to the animal nature.

These three consequences will be reviewed, in reverse order, in the following three chapters of this text. First, we will verify this separation of human and animal, and how the Lacanian conception of subjectivity runs counter to those experiments that attempt to measure, 'objectively,' the self-recognition of dolphins (and other species). Then, we will consider what relationship the erotogenic zones that fragment the body have with the aggressiveness that lies at the very birth of subjectivity, and how this fragmentation is fed by a contemporary phenomenon of the digital: the *selfie*. Lastly, we will consider this mediation of subjectivity through the desire of the other in a contemporary psychologized phenomenon: the liberal left so-called 'woke' movement, and its curious relation to (neoliberal) labor psychology.

Notes

1 For Spanish readers, we could say that *Ich/moi/ego* should be translated as "mi/yo" and *self* should be translated as "mi/yo mismo"—for example, "I saw myself" is "*me ví a mí mismo.*" It should be noted that Freud always talks about *Ich*, and if it could be extreme to say that Freud has *no* theoretical discussion on a concept that should be translated as "self" *and not as* "ego," it is certainly quite dubious

that he cared for it as much as he cared for the *Ich*/ego. It is difficult to find a reference for the German *Selbst* in Freud, apart from its uses in the sense of an action of the ego directed towards itself (e.g., he talks about "self-analysis" [*Selbstanalyse*] in Freud 1957/XI, p. 145), or as a word simply emphasizing an object (e.g., "[a] portion of the lip itself" [*Lippe selbst*] in Freud, 1953/VII, p. 180). I think that the conditions to start talking about a possible 'Freudian theory of the self' (in contraposition to the ego) should start addressing the issue of translation, and I don't think that is the usual way this discussion starts.

2 In the text *Presentation on Psychical Causality*, Lacan explains this idea as follows: "the subject identifies, in his feeling of Self, with the other's image and that the other's image captivates this feeling in him" (Lacan, 1966, p. 147). A curious and not-so-much commented anticipation of this Lacanian idea was in a footnote by Freud, in 1920's *Beyond the Pleasure Principle* (1955/XVIII), just after explaining the meaning of *fort* (gone) and *Da* (here) in the trolley game: "A further observation subsequently confirmed this interpretation fully. One day the child's mother had been away for several hours and on her return was met with the words 'Baby o-o-o-o!' which was at first incomprehensible. It soon turned out, however, that during this long period of solitude the child had found a method of making *himself* disappear. He had discovered his reflection in a full-length mirror which did not quite reach to the ground, so that by crouching down he could make his mirror-image 'gone'" (Freud, 1955/XVIII, p. 15). The child had succeeded in using his own image as an object in the world.

3 Again, *Presentation on Psychical Causality*: "the first effect of the imago that appears in human beings is that of the subject's *alienation*. It is in the other that the subject first identifies himself and even experiences himself" (Lacan, 1966, p. 148).

4 This idea, "a subjective synthesis in objective terms," offers us a definition of *psychologization*: psychologizing therapies and discourses try to objectify subjectivity, to offer a succinct and precise explanation, via their tools of objectification, of human subjectivity. More on this in the discussion on the applications of labor psychology.

5 It is because of this condition, in addition to motor incapacity, that Lacan speaks of "a veritable *specific prematurity of birth*" in the human individual (p. 78).

6 Few things are as clear about this as that popular idea that, as a Mexican popular saying goes, "dessert does not go to the stomach, but to the heart": precisely what is indicated here is that no matter whether the biological need for hunger has been satisfied (which is always achieved before dessert), there is something *extra* that is always welcome for *pleasure that goes beyond satisfaction*.

7 The literal translation is "the drop that overflowed the arm... sorry, the glass," which comes from the popular saying "la gota que derramó el vaso." The English version is "the straw that broke the camel's back." Perhaps, a translation of her lapsus could be "the straw that broke the camel's lack... sorry, back."

8 An essential place to understand the consequences of this psychoanalytic approach to human subjectivity is the work of Jan de Vos, especially, for this issue in particular, *Psychologization and the Subject of Late Modernity* (2013).

9 Why, then, are memes so popular? We can point out one path from a psychoanalytic standpoint: because they aim at a reinforcement of the self, via identifying it with an object, a position or a situation, even in spite of making fun of it. At times when we reproach our own stupidity, we can locate that something is knotted in the fact of *identifying* the stupidity itself, as when we are embarrassed by our own laughter, and the attempt to hide it seems to inflate our desire to laugh even more.

10 Many years later, when I read Freud for the first time (it was *The Uncanny*), I had an uncanny (!) feeling when I read that Freud had a very similar anecdote in a train (1955/XVII, footnote on p. 248).

References

De Vos, Jan. (2013). *Psychologization and the Subject of Late Modernity.* Palgrave Macmillan.

Freud, Sigmund. [1895] (1966). "Project for a Scientific Psychology." In *The Standard Edition of The Complete Psychological Works of Sigmund Freud*, Vol. I. The Hogarth Press, pp. 281–397.

Freud, Sigmund. [1910] (1957). "The Future Prospects of Psycho-Analytic Therapy." In *The Standard Edition of The Complete Psychological Works of Sigmund Freud*, Vol. XI. The Hogarth Press, pp. 139–151.

Freud, Sigmund. [1905] (1953). "Three Essays on the Theory of Sexuality." In *The Standard Edition of The Complete Psychological Works of Sigmund Freud*, Vol. VII. The Hogarth Press, pp. 124–254.

Freud, Sigmund. [1919] (1955). "The 'Uncanny'." In *The Standard Edition of The Complete Psychological Works of Sigmund Freud*, Vol. XVII. The Hogarth Press, pp. 217–256.

Freud, Sigmund. [1920] (1955). "Beyond the Pleasure Principle." In *The Standard Edition of The Complete Psychological Works of Sigmund Freud*, Vol. XVIII. The Hogarth Press, pp. 1–64.

Lacan, Jacques. [1936] (2006). "Beyond the 'Reality Principle'." In *Écrits. The First Complete Edition in English.* W.W. Norton & Company, pp. 58–74.

Lacan, Jacques. [1946] (2006). "Presentation on Psychical Causality." In *Écrits. The First Complete Edition in English.* W.W. Norton & Company, pp. 123–158.

Lacan, Jacques. [1949] (2006). "The Mirror Stage as Formative of the *I* Function as Revealed in Psychoanalytic Experience." In *Écrits. The First Complete Edition in English.* W.W. Norton & Company, pp. 75–81.

4

ANIMALS AND THE LACANIMAL

The first consequence of the mirror stage is the radical separation of human subjectivity from any kind of animal nature. A common fantasy of the contemporary world is the attempt to return us to our 'animality' in the constant reminder that *we are animals*: from neuroscience that reduces us to our 'mirror neurons,' to business *coaching* that compares the logics of neoliberal exploitation with an 'evolution' or 'triumph of the best adapted,' to the animalistic discourses that equate puppy dogs with human babies. For his part, during the 1950s and 1960s, Lacan had an interesting preoccupation with animality, especially because from animals he could locate the complex relationship that sustains the human animal (i.e., the *subject*) and the *other*, as well as the alienation of the subject from any supposed 'animal nature.'

From the mirror test to the mirror stage

It was from the question of the distinction between humans and animals that Lacan, at the beginning of his work, located several ways of understanding the constitutive split of the subject. As a matter of fact, Lacan was highly interested in using animals to explain, deepen and question many essential moments of his teaching.[1] For example, in Seminar 1 (1953–1954), chronologically close to *The Mirror Stage*, the split is one between the biological organism studied by anatomy and the body given to us by the other (in the lesson of May 5, 1954):

> The image of the other's form is assumed by the subject. Thanks to this surface, situated within the subject, what is introduced into human psychology is this relation between the outside and the inside whereby the subject knows himself, gets acquainted with himself as body.

DOI: 10.4324/9781003640653-4

> Besides, it is the sole truly fundamental difference between human and animal psychology. Man knows himself as body, whereas there is, after all, no reason why he should know himself, since he is inside it. The animal is also inside it, but we have no reason for thinking that he represents it to himself.
>
> *(Lacan, [1954] 1988, p. 170)*

Thus, the difference between human psychology and animal psychology is not established on the basis of the organic differences of the brain, but on the basis of a knowledge about itself: for Lacan, on this point, the difference between the animal and the human is that we know that we have a body and that we know that—that is, we have a direct relation to our bodies (we have one) and a reflexive relation (we *know* that we have one). In the case of the animal, we have no guarantee that this also applies: do animals know that they *have a body*? Do animals have a reflexive relation to their own body?

It is here that we return to the dolphin experiment, mentioned in the Introduction. This experiment, which became fashionable with primates in the 1970s and has since been verified with other animals (such as magpies, elephants and pigs) is known in zoology as *the mirror test*, and basically the mechanism is the same among species: mark the animals in a place where they cannot see the mark except with a mirror, and verify their behavior in front of it.

According to the authors of one of these experiments (Plotnik, de Waal & Reiss, 2006, p. 17053) done with Asian elephants (*Elephas maximus*), if the animals successfully pass the test, it is because they go through four stages: (1) a "social response" (i.e., the animal behaves before the mirror image as it behaves when it sees another of its own species); (2) "physical mirror inspection" (i.e., it checks the mirror's material and what lies behind and beside it); (3) "repetitive mirror-testing behavior" (i.e., movements it makes before the mirror over and over again); and the last, certainly the most problematic, (4) "self-directed behavior (i.e., recognition of the mirror image as self)." One soon notices the problem with these four stages: while the first three make a description of animal *behavior*, the fourth stage makes an assumption of *cognitive* processes in the animal, as their explanation in parenthesis implies—that is, in stages 1, 2 and 3, we simply see what the animal does; in stage 4, *we assume* what the animal *thinks*, for it is no longer a simple behavior, but a *recognition of self*.

In a similar experiment with the common magpie (*Pica pica*), its authors summarize, in other words, the interests of these experiments:

> If an individual is experimentally provided with a mark that cannot be directly seen but is, however, visible in the mirror, increased exploration of the own body and self-directed actions towards the mark suggest that the mirror image is being perceived as self.
>
> *(Prior, Schwarz & Güntürkün, 2008, p. 0001)*

This paragraph introduces us in a mix of concepts. The word "self," presented twice, is introduced both to speak of animal actions directed to the body ("self-directed actions") and as an assumption that animals perceive themselves in the body ("perceived as self"). What the zoologists performing these experiments too quickly conclude is that *self-directed* and *perceived as self* are equally evident, equally measurable, equally verifiable. It seems that zoologists have no problem in assuming what the animal 'knows' or 'thinks.'

In the presentation of the methodology of the dolphin experiment (Reiss & Marino, 2001, p. 5397), the authors point out that they worked with dolphins born in captivity—that is, animals that have spent more time with humans than with different members of their own species; however, they never question how the fact that these animals have spent more time with humans than with members of their own species comes into play. Above this, a more fundamental question: what was it that the mark *marked* the dolphin? Did the dolphin know that the mark was on *its* body? What prevents us from thinking that the dolphin saw the mark as something that was in the mirror? What prevents us from thinking that the dolphin saw the mark as something that was on the body of another dolphin? What prevents us from thinking that the dolphin saw the mirror image as its own double, as if it were a science fiction movie? Or how can we know that the dolphins did not experience a moment of psychic dissociation, as happens with those who experiment with acid drugs or those who have psychotic breaks, not knowing if it was on their body or just imagining it was there?

When we see these experiments and the conclusions reached by the scientists performing them, we cannot help but wonder how zoologists know that, for example, the magpie knows that it is seeing the reflection of its body or rather believes that it is seeing another magpie, so that perhaps it is not trying to remove his mark but is checking whether it does not have on its body the mark that it sees that *another magpie* in front of it. It could be objected that if this were the case, then they would do similar things when they see other magpies with strange marks on their bodies to what they do in front of a mirror, but, again, how do we know what magpies would do if they saw another magpie with a strange mark? Why do we assume that magpies would 'do something' if they saw that there was a mark on their body or on another magpie's body?

In the case of the elephants, let's assume that the elephant passed the test and 'recognizes its self in the mirror,' as the researchers conclude (Plotnik, de Waal and Reiss, 2006, p. 17054). So, the elephant recognizes its image, but does it know its body as *its body*? Does the elephant, as the human subject, have a problem of correspondence between its body and the self, or in terms of our discussion, *between body and the ego*? Do elephants have anorexic or bulimic behaviors, so that seeing the ribs on their body or feeling the burning of acid in their throat, they insist that they are fat or that they should vomit? Do elephants, when mating, have love triangles and ambivalent feelings towards their partner? Do elephants have sexual fetishes regarding the body of the elephant they mate with? It is a radical matter: I cannot claim that they do *not* comply with this, but it is clear to me that *we can never know*, for our isolation from animals is more radical. It is not that we are a 'superior' species in intelligence, but that language has left us in a radical isolation from other animals that is evidenced in these delusions of the 'self' of elephants.[2]

Let us return to the quote from Seminar 1. For Lacan, there is no clear difference between animals and humans, but not because of an 'anti-speciesism' bet or a 'pro-animal' activism, but because we simply do not have the elements to verify that difference: we do not know how animals pose themselves against us or other animals, as, precisely, we distinguish *us* and *other animals*. We can say, for example, that dolphins recognize a diversity of animals (them, humans, orcas, fish and other animals), but we do not know if they recognize *a difference between themselves and all other animals.*

The discourses that attempt to reduce human experience to its animal condition try to disavow this radical impossibility, offering some account that tries to 'demonstrate' that we are animals. From the side of zoosemiotics, and returning to birds, zoologist Carles Riba (1990, p. 112[3]) comments that, if a bird specialist can recognize different birds just by listening to them, we can suppose that birds also recognize different human voices. Anyone who has owned a parrot knows this, but we should ask ourselves whether birds, like us, hear voices in the middle of the night as when we watch a horror movie, whether they hear things different from what we are told in a Freudian slip, or whether their very precise songs admit equivocity through homophonies, as when we hear lyrics in a song differently from how the artist wrote it. The bird has *a body that produces sounds*, but we do not know if it admits *the voice as an object*, as something foreign to itself that comes from within (as I mentioned above about listening to our own recorded voice), which is for humans an instance where the estrangement between the body and the ego is evident.

From a deceiving deception to a truthful deception

Animals allow us to continue verifying this split between the ego and the body that Lacan speaks of. Let us consider another example, now taken from Seminar 10 (1962–1963), where an interesting discussion on the falsity and erasure of traces is established (in the lesson of December 5, 1962):

> Animals, I tell you, efface their traces and lay false traces. Do they for all that make signifiers? There's one thing that animals don't do—they don't lay false traces to make us believe that they are false, that is, traces that will be taken for false. Laying falsely false traces is a behaviour that is, I won't say quintessentially human, but quintessentially signifying. That's where the limit is. That's where a subject presentifies himself. When a

> trace has been made to be taken for a false trace, though in fact they are the traces of my true passage, we know that there's a subject as cause.
>
> *(Lacan, [1962] 2014, p. 63)*

In the traces that I make so that the other believes that they are false when they are true is where I evidence my condition as subject of language. How to understand this?

Let us think that Lacan is referring to different types of deception. The first type is *simple deception*: one deceives by making the other believe that a thing is X when in reality it is Y. Clearly, this is the deception that works in the animal world: the alligator snapping turtle (*Macrochelys temminckii*) has a protrusion on its tongue that looks like a worm; when fish come to eat it, the turtle eats them: one deceives and the other is deceived.

The second type of deception is *disguise*: one presents oneself to the other as X, when both one and the other know that in reality it is Y, and both one and the other know that both know that it is a disguise, so that it is not a deceit, but a simulation: when we go to a costume party where someone has dressed up as Freud or a turtle, we know that it is not Freud or a turtle, but a *disguise* of Freud or a turtle, and the disguised person knows that we know that this is a disguise. This second deception, perhaps, is also encountered among animals: Riba (1990, pp. 149–150) tells us of rites where male apes hold a "false copulation" because their buttocks look similar to those of females, and this "wrong" signal is perfectly incorporated as an "accepted deception" within the group of apes.[4]

The third deception, the *signifying deception*, is what Lacan says is proper to the human subject: it consists in one presenting X in such a way that the other believes it is a deception (say, he believes it is Y disguised as X), when in fact there is no deception, for it *is* X. Cinema offers us a very powerfully explicit scene of this: the first sequence of *The Dark Knight* (dir. Christopher Nolan, 2008), a bank robbery performed by robbers with clown masks, betraying each other in order to get all the money for a smaller group. In the end, when only one clown is left, he shows his face to the bank manager: he is a clown (the main villain of the movie). The mask was presented as a deception, as something to be taken as 'not the true face,' when, actually, *it is his true face*: as a matter of fact, one of the interesting things in that movie is that we never know the Joker's name or who he 'actually' is.[5]

The signifying deception is *a deception that deceives in its condition of deception*: here, it is evident how human language does not allow us to sustain an objective relation with the truth, but that this is always subjectively mediated, so that there is no truth that is not *always already* crossed by the subject involved in it, not by what is said (the statement), but by the very act of saying it, hearing it or being involved in it (the enunciation).[6] We do not know if the animal sustains a relationship with the world that surrounds it in the same way that we sustain it with the truth that surrounds us, where a gap opens up between the statement and the enunciation.

From the rat that learns to the rat caught

One last place to grasp the decentering that the human subject introduces into the animal world: the very fact of simply observing this world constitutes a *hominization* of the world (as we shall see in a moment).

In Seminar 20 (1972–1973), Lacan wondered how we can conclude that rat-units "learn" through experiments that seek, precisely, to know if they learn. He tells us (in the lesson of June 26, 1973), in regard to experiments where rats press a button at the end of a maze:

> The only thing the rat-unit learns in this case is to give a sign, a sign of its presence as unit. The flap is recognized only by a sign and pressing its paw on this sign is a sign. It is always by making a sign that the unit accedes to that on the basis of which one concludes that there is learning. But this relation to signs is external. Nothing confirms that the rat grasps the mechanism to which pressing the button leads. That's why the only thing that counts is to know if the experimenter notes that the rat has not only figured it out, but learned (*appris*) how a mechanism is to be grasped (*se prend*), in other words, learned what must be grasped (*a-prendre*).
>
> *(Lacan, [1973] 1998, p. 141)*

The Lacanian play between "learned" and "grasped," as shown by the translator leaving those French words, is key here: before we could say anything about what *the rat has learned* (*appris*), we should consider how *the rat is grasped* (*a-prendre*) in the experiment. That is why he talks about a "rat-unit," for we consider the body and the interiority of the rat as one unit, quite contrary to what the human experience is in regard to the break between the body and the ego.[7]

But if this is the way things are, do such experiments really prove anything? Zoologists, in their attempt to understand animal behavior, do not hesitate to bring certain assumptions to the foundation of their observation: again, it is Riba who evidences this series of assumptions on which animal behavior is studied, such as the possibility that a human researcher is a mere "third party" excluded from that which he observes:

> The human observer must work based on the postulate of the universality of signification (a genuinely Peircian postulate). Man can receive information directly from an animal, but its optimal and usual position insofar a scientist shall be that of a "third party" situated in front of the interaction of two individuals from a species different from its own.
>
> *(Riba, 1990, p. 86)*

This bid to consider the position of the third party as optimal for the study of the animal interaction is on which Riba's *metalanguage* proposal is based (later on p. 86): the attempt to be able to speak about the animal's communication from an exteriority to the very subject that speaks of that communication. This is why Riba argues that *the animal is a subject* (p. 112–113, p. 191): his understanding of 'animal subject' is based on the fantasy of being able to speak of the animal subject and the human subject from a position of thirdness, which is why he can only speak of zoosemiotics from behaviorism[8]: thus, the possibility to speak about animal communication is grounded on the (not-so-explicit) assumption that we are talking about *animal behaviorist communication*.

Faced with this pretension of a thirdness alien to the subject that enunciates it, we should insist on a fundamental Lacanian question: is it really total exteriority, or only an exteriority possible under an assumption of disavowing our implication in its enunciation? Riba says that when we are observers of an exchange of communication between animals, "we continue receiving messages, even though these are not intentionally addressed to us. The 'third party' who observes [...] is condemned to observe significations, only that these, naturally, are not intended for him" (p. 87).

They are not intended for him, but the observer assumes that it *is still receiving messages*; that is, the observer is involved in the animal exchange even in his attempt not to be involved. It is curious that although he devotes a whole chapter in his book to criticize 'anthropocentrism,' Riba assumes that the human who observes the animal exchange is also someone to whom messages are addressed, a 'subject' who can 'decipher' *the message addressed to him by the animals, even if it is not intentionally addressed.*

From nonhuman to inhuman to post-human

The mirror stage, then, presents us with our radical separation from any account of a 'primordial' human animality, or any attempt to return to a 'natural' animality. Unlike, on the one hand, cognitive-behaviorism that claims that animals use semiotic codes just as we do, and, on the other hand, holistic and 'anti-speciesist' activism that insists on affirming an animality that can only be affirmed through human language, psychoanalysis maintains an irreducible gap between the body and the ego of the human subject.

Other biologist discourses pretend to study the human being as one more animal that populates the planet, regardless of its complexity. However, these approaches are not free from certain psychologizing assumptions that implicitly indicate what kind of understanding of humans they have in order to study them as *other animals.* For these endeavors, behaviorism is an important ally, for behavioral psychology has, at its foundations, psychological presuppositions that are expressed in the *measurable* behavior of the species: it is not for nothing that the foundation of comparative psychology (e.g., in the study of human and animal development) is precisely *behaviorism*, and their findings are impacting in multiple contemporary applications, from brief psychotherapy to educational models.

Nonetheless, we should ask: what kind of concept does behaviorism have of the *animal*, and what kind of reductions does this imply for our understanding of the *human subject*? Those discourses that we pour over animals, their behavior and—with greater delirium—their 'thinking' are only attempts to continue, narcissistically, to impose the human *imago* on the objects of the world.

This is what Lacan referred to in the early text *Beyond the "Reality Principle"* of 1936, when he pointed out that nature is shaped as myth precisely at the moment when we point out that we are part of nature:

> In any case, man's idea of a world that is united to him through a harmonious relationship allows us to divine its basis in the anthropomorphism of the myth of *nature*. As the effort is achieved that animates this idea, the reality of this basis is revealed in the ever vaster subversion of nature implied by the *hominization* of the planet: the "nature" of man is its relationship to man.
>
> *(Lacan, 1966, p. 70–71)*

What to make of this "*hominization* of the planet"? Are we animals or are we not animals? For psychoanalysis, the problem is not *where* the division between animals and humans is, but in realizing that *the difference itself*, in its zero degree, is what constitutes the human.

Another way to put it is that the key division is between what is human and that which is *inhuman*: only human beings inhabit an inhuman dimension. For Žižek (2012, p. 166), the line that distinguishes the *nonhuman* from the *inhuman* is evident: the *nonhuman* is simply that thing that *is not human*, like the computer on which I am writing this, or the sun shining through a window, or the dog walking down the street; on the other hand, the *inhuman* is something that has crossed humanity: it is something that we think of as nonhuman *and* that is only possible insofar as it *is* human. Animals kill other animals, but they do not make concentration camps with them, nor do they look for more 'effective' methods to kill them. Animals have sex, but they do not produce pornography or sexually exploit others of their species. Animals eat, but they do not have eating contests, nor do they suffer from anorexia or bulimia. We can without much difficulty think of inhuman actions committed by humans, because only humans can commit inhuman acts, but we cannot think of 'incanine' or 'infeline' actions, because dogs and cats are not decentered from themselves; they do not commit acts excessive towards a Symbolic line that defines the limits of their actions and that point to a split in their subjectivity, no matter how wild, aggressive or beastly they may seem to us.[9]

It is possible that some might think to object to this position from the 'post-anthropocentric turn.' The problem with imagining any 'post-anthropocentric' state is that we can only do so from an anthropocentric standpoint: that is the trap of the hominization of the planet that Lacan pointed out in the last quote. A final example to think about this is the 2024 animated film *Flow* (dir. Gints Zilbalodis): the story of a cat and a group of animals trying to survive an inhospitable world that is being intermittently flooded.

The film opens with the cat seeing itself in a reflection, like a mirror returning his image. A gregarious instinct runs through all the animals in the film, and even among a biological diversity, *the animals live together* in a boat. There is, however, an animal that has an ambivalent function in the plot: a whale that, with monstrous proportions and appendages on its body, seems at times to be helping the protagonists and at times trying to kill them.

Towards the end of the film, after the flood has subsided and the animals find relative tranquility, the cat encounters the whale. At this point, there is a sequence of glances interchanged between the cetacean and the feline, but something particular happens: the only moment in the entire film where we have a detail shot of an eye, where an eye occupies the entire screen, is with the whale.

There is a curious function of this shot: unlike several close-ups in the film, where we see the animal reacting to something that happens in its environment, here we see the whale seeing; as if far from being a reaction to the cat in front of it, the key point in this shot is that *it is seeing*. What is important is not what it sees, but the fact that it is seeing, and to a large extent, this gaze is not only looking at us: it is because the whale/the gaze is us. The whale in *Flow* represents the human gaze in the film (the whale among the animals) and towards the film (in a more abstract dimension, the gaze *in* the film is the gaze *of* the film). The whale's gaze is the correlate of the human gaze on animals, a gaze that is in constant alienation with them: the whale cannot live if the animals live; they cannot live if it lives. The whale, although it is an animal, is an animal whose existence is at disjunction with the other animals, who look at it with awe and fear. The whale returns them an unsettling gaze, but, at the same time, a helpless one: it is dying at that moment.

Thus, what we find at the end of *Flow* is a reflection of our own gaze. The film is anything but 'post-anthropocentric': the final point of the film is that the fantasy of a 'post-anthropocene' is only in the human gaze that constructs that fantasy. It is not a coincidence that the musical piece playing during that sequence is called *Reflection*, an ambivalent word: it implies both a reflection in a mirror and a reflection of our subjective position. Our *reflection* in *Flow*'s whale contains the dimension of the image (what the mirror returns) as well as the imago (the assumption of that image). Our relationship with animals and with our animality is crossed by an impossibility of direct transparency: we are (not) animals.

These three splits within the human (between body and ego; between deceiving and being deceived; between simple observation and involvement in what is observed) lead us to consider that, for psychoanalysis, the split within the human is a constitutive split of itself: the human subject is such because it cannot be *totally as such*. In other words, although the human *is* an animal, it is certainly an animal in whom animality is a *problem*: what distinguishes the human from other animals is that it is *an animal for whom its animality is problematic*, inasmuch as it is inhabited by an irreducible gap between its body and its ego. The name for that gap is *subject*, the Lacanimal *par excellence.*

While we see a dolphin, an elephant, a magpie and a cat as animals that *are* dolphins, elephants, magpies and cats, we notice that the decentering produced by the subject makes the human an animal that is *like* a human. What defines the human being is precisely its name, where we find the necessary doubleness to affirm itself: the human *being* is a continuous attempt *to be* a human.

Notes

1 A complete tour through the animals that appear in Lacan's work is given by Macola & Brandalise (2006), although with somewhat different purposes than those of this chapter.
2 This isolation is not perceived by scientists, who do not even hesitate to assume what the elephants' canons of *beauty* and self-care are towards themselves, or to assume that an elephant understands pouring mud on its body as getting it *dirty* (Plotnik, de Waal and Reiss, 2006, p. 17055).
3 All translations from Spanish sources are mine.
4 How he knows that apes engage in *false* copulation and not simply *homosexual* copulation is not clearly explained by Riba.
5 Todd Phillips' *Joker* (2019) made an homage to this sequence in a scene that we could also use as an example, when Arthur Fleck escapes the policeman by putting a clown mask over his clown costume in the subway scene.
6 This was indicated by Freud in regard to the joke of the two Jews traveling by train (in 1960/VIII, p. 63).
7 And also very important: what kind of "learning" is considered to take place because a rat pushes a button, and how do these conclusions support the 'learning theories' that schools have today? We do not know then *what* the rat "learned", nor *how* the rat positions itself with respect to its learning, just as we maintain a reflexivity with respect to our own learning process.
8 Let us not forget that John Watson, considered the father of behaviorism, was an animal psychologist interested in moving towards the objectification of human psychology. With his ideas on behaviorism, which Lacan criticizes in several texts of the 1950s, he sought to create a doctrine that excludes any approach to psychism. These models are the foundation of the incorporation of psychology in American universities, and due to the academic imperialism of the world, it is what is standardized to consider a 'scientific psychology.' For an introduction to the figure of Watson, behaviorism and its applications, see chapter 11 of Leahey's history of psychology (2018).
9 Todd McGowan's great piece (2018) is dedicated to deepening this idea through the insults we say to each other that use animal similes.

References

Freud, Sigmund. [1905] (1960). "Jokes and their Relation to the Unconscious." In *The Standard Edition of The Complete Psychological Works of Sigmund Freud*, Vol. VIII. The Hogarth Press.

Lacan, Jacques. [1936] (2006). "Beyond the 'Reality Principle'." In *Écrits. The First Complete Edition in English*. W.W. Norton & Company, pp. 58–74.

Lacan, Jacques. [1953–1954] (1988). *The Seminar of Jacques Lacan. Book I. Freud's Papers on Technique*. W.W. Norton & Company.

Lacan, Jacques. [1962–1963] (2014). *Anxiety. The Seminar of Jacques Lacan. Book X*. Polity.

Lacan, Jacques. [1972–1973] (1998). *The Seminar of Jacques Lacan. Book XX. Encore*. W.W. Norton & Company.

Leahey, Thomas Hardy. (2018). *A History of Psychology: From Antiquity to Modernity* (8th edition). Routledge.

Macola, Erminia & Brandalise, Adone. (2006). *Bestiario lacaniano*. Miguel Gómez Ediciones.

McGowan, Todd. (2018). "Like an Animal: A Simile Instead of a Subject." In Gautam Basu Thakur & Jonathan Michael Dickstein (eds.). *Lacan and the Non-human*. Palgrave Macmillan, pp. 177–198.

Plotnik, Joshua M., de Waal, Frans B. M. & Reiss, Diana. (2006). "Self-recognition in an Asian elephant." *Proceedings of the National Academy of Sciences of the United States of America*, Vol. 103, No. 45, pp. 17053–17057.

Prior, Helmut, Schwarz, Ariane & Güntürkün, Onur. (2008). "Mirror-Induced Behavior in the Magpie (*Pica pica*): Evidence of Self-Recognition." *PLoS Biology*, Vol. 6, No. 8, pp. 1–9.

Reiss, Diana & Marino, Lori. (2001). "Mirror self-recognition in the bottlenose dolphin: A case of cognitive convergence." *Proceedings of the National Academy of Sciences of the United States of America*, Vol. 98, No. 10, pp. 5937–5942.

Riba, Carles. (1990). *La comunicación animal. Un enfoque zoosemiótico*. Anthropos.

Žižek, Slavoj. (2012). *Less than Nothing*. Verso.

5

THE FRAGMENTED SELF AND ITS SELFIE

The second consequence of the mirror stage is that aggressiveness against the other is a constitutive dimension of one's own fragmented subjectivity. What kind of subjectivity results in a subject who is burdened with a constitutive split between its body and the ego? I have pointed out the importance that Freud noted in what he called erotogenic zones, those which, due to their use for the satisfaction of a biological need, are charged with a kind of libidinization or extra pleasure: the satisfaction of the satisfaction itself is experienced as something that causes pleasure, and whose repetition is sought by the organ itself, in a manner alien and insensitive to the will of the ego. The subject, Lacan tells us in *The Mirror Stage* (p. 78), is trapped between his own organs that seek pleasure outside his interest, a "fragmented image of the body," and an artificial and alienating imago, an "'orthopedic' form of its totality," an identity which pretends to give the subject a failed sense of unity.

This introduces a certain disorder into the human body, caused by the erotogenization of its parts, in which each one has a life almost of its own: this part of the body is less than the whole body, but it is also excessive towards the body (as in the case of the woman with the arm/glass mentioned in a previous chapter). Lacan locates here the work of Hieronymus Bosch (p. 78) as a painter specialized in exposing the living fragmentation of the body: an ear with a knife, a smiling head and a foot protruding from a fruit are some of the characters that populate his famous *The Garden of Earthly Delights* (1515).

This fragmentation of the body, and, more precisely, the fascination it seems to produce in how we relate to this type of image, is something that Lacan considered essential in the relationship between one's subjectivity and aggressiveness towards the other.

DOI: 10.4324/9781003640653-5

From the hostile other to snuff images

Works like Bosch's are correlative to a certain contemporary fascination, quite uncanny, with violent images: from snuff images, hardcore pornography, videos of skateboarder accidents and images of babies born with deformities to those circulated by terrorist groups, from the Islamic State to Los Zetas. The image of a bleeding head, a hand separated from the body or genitals being mutilated constitute not only images showing this or that, but also imagos, more specifically, "imagos of the fragmented body" (p. 85), as Lacan defines them in *Aggressiveness in Psychoanalysis* (originally from 1948) which "represent the elective vectors of aggressive intentions, which they provide with an efficacy that might be called magical" (p. 85).

Why do these images repulse us and at the same time attract us with "an efficacy that might be called magical"? Despite showing only a specific part of the body, these images carry a hyperlibidinization that stains the whole image, as if that part of the body had a life that runs parallel to that of the rest of the organism.

In the case of pornography, this is very evident: we might assume that it is not until genitalia and penetration are explicitly shown that a film ceases to be highly erotic and becomes pornography. Such is pornography's obsession with hyperlibidinization of genitalia that there are even videos showing the ejaculation of a penis from inside a sex toy.

In the case of snuff images, where tortured, mutilated, dismembered bodies are shown, an escape route is offered for a certain aggressive intention of the subject, which cannot be channeled openly due to cultural restraints: is there no more obvious representation of this idea than the photos of Abu Ghraib, *protoselfies* where U.S. soldiers mock the tortures to which they subject their political prisoners while smiling at the camera? It should be obvious to us that what is particularly shocking about these images is not the acts presented, but precisely that *they are images of those acts*: as Naief Yehya (2013, p. 218) points out, similar or worse tortures and mockeries have been known about in other war conflicts, but the specific quality of the Abu Ghraib photos was their pornographic quality—that is, the fact that *their materiality as digital images* produced in the public an open repugnance (the official version of the U.S. military was that they were just 'bad elements') *and* a hidden fascination (as they involved images that in the traditional media were only alluded to or harshly censored, while they circulated on violent pornography websites).

Museum montages could serve as a snuff libidinization in this sense. The concentration camp facilities in Auschwitz are quite a good example of this: in them, we can find pools filled with objects that belonged to the political prisoners who ended up there, from suitcases and cans of food to shoes, toys and many other belongings. One that particularly stands out is the one filled with human hair. The superficial reading indicates that these installations are to 'raise awareness' of the dimensions of the tragedy of the Holocaust, to 'never forget' about what happened, and while this is true, one must also note the power of fascination exerted by these pools of bodily fragmentation: it would seem that the hair of the dead has a life of its own, and that the power of subjective impact on museum visitors is due to a condition of hyperlibidinization. That is to say, the conclusion that imposes itself is that this 'conscientization' is only achieved with a libidinous spectacularization, with a kind of unconscious enjoyment of this fragment of the body. The final scenes of Jonathan Glazer's *The Zone of Interest* (2023) exposes this paradox of a quiet place that, on the surface, has a function of remembering the victims, but also functions as a place of enjoyment, even if it is a guilt we assume when seeing hundreds of faces in photographs: the fact that those places are shown while being cleaned by women, just like the women serving in the house of Rudolf Höss and his family through the movie, makes us question if couldn't it be that the price to pay in order to 'never forget' the Holocaust is to still work for the Nazis.

This aggressiveness is not strange to psychoanalysis; on the contrary, it seems to be a *sine qua non* condition of human subjectivity. Let us recall that, in the *Project*, Freud placed the *fellow human-being* as an object that, besides being similar to the ego, "simultaneously the [subject's] first satisfying object and further his first hostile object, as well as his sole helping power" (Freud, 1966/I, p. 331). The fellow human is the first object of satisfaction because it calms my hunger, gives me warmth to sleep, cleans me of my bodily waste; but it is also a hostile object because it does not always give me what I ask for, either by denying me or giving me something I do not want, when not directly attacking me. The child becomes aware that the other does not always have the answer; that the other denies me what I want and, therefore, is hostile to me. An aggressiveness against the other has been formed, on which the human being learns to discern between itself and the other, between its self and the other's.

Because we contain much more aggressiveness against others than we express, we need a process of canalization of that excessive aggressiveness, and we find it, among other places and ways, in the scopic and auditory satisfaction of these kinds of violent material, of seeing and hearing them. These images work to help satisfy a sort of inclination towards aggressiveness, which is exhibited since childhood and finds a correlate in children's games: breaking a doll, throwing objects from a height, the obsession with fire and other acts that infants constantly manifest and that even creep into their stories, where the children themselves are imprisoned or devoured by witches or monsters. There is a curious fascination in children for those sadistic acts that we continue as adults, when we make bad and humiliating jokes to our closest friends, jokes that we would not make to those we are just beginning to know or who we do not consider someone close, because, after all, is not a way to notice the closeness and trust that someone has towards us in the fact that they openly mock us, that they process some of their aggressiveness towards us precisely to continue the good relationship they have with us?

Lacan brings the important conclusion that this ambivalence of the other, the fact that the other "is simultaneously the first object-satisfaction and the first hostile object" (as Freud says, 1966/I, p. 331), points to a fundamental role aggressiveness has in the birth of subjectivity, that these images where the subject processes its aggressiveness have a "formative function" in itself (Lacan, 1966, p. 85).

It is this fundamental aggressiveness in human subjectivity that does not allow psychoanalysis to so easily believe that dialogue is a simple bridge to unite the individuals: rather, dialogue is an attempt, often more unsuccessful than successful, to control that aggressiveness that the self feels towards the other. Aggressiveness is not only the current state of civilization, but also its foundation, and it plays an essential role in its current state.[1]

Thus, the conformation of the ego, and of its *self* as the main imago that the ego uses to interact with others, cannot but pass through an ambivalent function, of satisfaction and hostility from and towards the other.[2] This erection of a self *in relation to the other* presupposes the "dialectic of identifications" (Lacan, 1966, p. 91). Through the body of the other, its face, the objects of its body (the breasts, the hands) and the objects that represent it (clothing, perfume, the bottle to feed me), the infant gradually configures the recognition of its own body as *an otherness for the other*; that is, the infant realizes that, just as the ego takes the other as an object, so the other takes the ego as an object. The consequence of this is then a certain transitivity in the infant, that *it is through the recognition of the other that I acquire a certain sense of self*: it is through getting to know the other that I get to know my/self. As we have seen many times with small children who fall during walking, they do not start crying until an adult recognizes their fall, so that if they fall and are ignored, they might not cry: I once heard someone tell the anecdote that he felt pretty badly on the street as a child, and walked back home, and it was not until he saw the concern of his family, when they saw his face full of blood, that he began to feel the pain of the fall. How can this cry be understood other than as *a call for the other to*, before healing the pain of the fall, *recognize my own pain*? How can it not be noticed that the pain of one's own body seems to need, at least sometimes, to pass through the expression of the other, so that I only feel the pain *in my body* until I can feel it *through the other*?

The selfie as image and distribution

A very precise place where we can recognize the imaginary construction of the self as a continuous, constant and hysterical call for the recognition of the other is the world of digital social media, and within it, perhaps no other manifestation evidences more clearly the fragmentation of the body and the constitution of the self/image for the other than the *selfie*. My interest in what follows is not only to expose the selfie as a phenomenon proper to the expansion of a hyperindividualist idea of a "sovereign self" (an idea I will expand in the next chapter), but to also criticize some approaches to it from communication and media studies.[3]

In his discussion of the topic, Naief Yehya (2013, p. 282) defines selfie as "a photo in which a person portrays her/himself in front of a mirror or by extending an arm to point a digital camera or the omnipresent cell phone cameras." In this definition, we find two points that distinguish the selfie from a portrait or self-portrait.

Unlike a portrait, which can be commissioned to another person acting as a photographer, (1) the selfie must be taken by the person who appears in it; and, unlike a self-portrait, (2) an essential condition in the selfie is that the subject must be seen in the image as participating in the very creation of the selfie, that the selfie shows how the selfie is being taken by the person portrayed (the famous arm extended beyond the frame of the image, the famous selfie stick that has precisely that purpose as an extension of the body, or the simple taking of the selfie in front of a mirror, so that the cell phone is visible). These two conditions, subtle and apparently insignificant, are important in considering a certain function that selfies have today: it is then an *image* in which *the self presents itself* and *shows* the conditions that procure this presentation. If we were to believe what certain ideas of 'media appropriation' might want us to believe, it becomes obvious how the subject then exposes his 'own' identity through the selfie.

However, there is something missing from Yehya's definition that subsequent studies on selfies (all those mentioned in the rest of this chapter agree on this) clearly indicate; for example, Clint Burnham (2018, p. 185), in his pages dedicated to this topic, states that the selfie "is marked by (is an event because of) being networked (shared), shot with a digital device ('handheld,' which then means touched), and made by the subject viewing their own image as part of making the image." As a matter of fact, it is precisely for this reason that Burnham considers that "the selfie offers new ways of thinking about Lacan's mirror stage" (p. 185).

The selfie is not simply the image itself or the conditions and dynamics under which it was taken, but, almost obviously and inherently, the *specific process of its distribution in digital social media*. In other words, the selfie is not a selfie if it is not distributed on digital social media.

We can think of the selfie as an image offered to the other. If the image that I have of myself has the intention of being sanctioned by the other, as the selfie does, for its purpose is not to be only a portrait but a portrait to be distributed, then the selfie is not only an exhibition of the self but, especially, *an exhibition of my/self to the other*. The selfie is not simply a 'spontaneous' expression of our subjectivity, but the *production of* an image of the self to be sanctioned by the *other*. That is why the phenomenon of the selfie is incomprehensible outside the digital media ecosystem that popularized it: the selfie is popular *because of* its capacity for instantaneousness in its production (the image on the cell phone) and circulation (in the networks to which this image is uploaded).

The selfie as a celebration

Just as a child, I pointed out earlier, starts crying after a fall only when the other has seen her/him fall, so a selfie only makes sense if it is circulating to be sanctioned by others. On several occasions, I have heard of people who have deleted a *selfie* from their Instagram account because it received few reactions or because it received mocking, unexpected or contrary reactions to those it was intended for. Moreover, this presentation to the other in itself is already an act, so that it does not matter what is shown, but the very fact that *something is being shown*: a banal and daily repeated walk down a street on the way to the supermarket or a Sunday family gathering become *events* (Murolo, 2015, p. 696) through their portrayal in a selfie.

Norberto Murolo distinguishes between the function of photographs as *a memory of the past* from the function of selfies as *a celebration of the present*. The former are photos of memorable moments, such as a wedding, a birthday, an important event in one's life; they are photographs that, when we take them, we assume that they will be seen in the future to remember the past. Selfies, on the contrary, are not usually of such memorable moments; in fact, most of them refer to those banal moments that become newsworthy for the simple fact of having been captured in a selfie: they are 'worthy' to remember only because they are in a selfie. This idea, undoubtedly very interesting, turns out to be poorly exploited, because from this intuition, Murolo ends up considering that the selfie responds to a "need" of the subject "to represent itself":

> "Why do we take selfies?", that would be a question pertinent to communication. To represent ourselves. The natural and the social subject has a need to represent itself. This need has to do with the experimentation of our own fears, with celebrating ourselves, with controlling as much as possible the image that others see of us. To represent ourselves is to present ourselves again within parameters of communicational construction that somehow control our uncertainty.
>
> *(Murolo, 2015, p. 696)*

It is never clear in his text what a "natural" and a "social" subject is, nor why the selfie satisfies the "need" of the subject to "represent itself." It would seem that the selfie is an 'obvious' or 'normal' way of "representing oneself," as if the selfie did not respond to certain technological practices that produce a certain type of subjectivity,[4] or as if that "need" came from an interiority not traversed by an otherness that sanctions it. As if this 'celebration' did not function under the conditions of the society of the spectacle: of reducing any attempt at celebration to a logic of capital reproduction (a theme we will encounter again in the next chapter).

Against accepting this idea of a 'need to represent oneself,' we must inquire whether the selfie is a result of the production of my/self for the other. It seems that Murolo begins to approach this point when referring to selfie representation as given "within the parameters of communicational construction," but he does not go to the ultimate consequences of this idea. Although he recognizes that this representation is given to be seen by the other, within the framework of certain parameters imposed by the other, he still considers that we *already* have an image of ourselves that is *then* "codified" for those parameters; whereas the point I am making is that even that 'self-image' is not really our own, just as the body we inhabit does not have a transparent relationship with our ego: that self-image is not born out of a subjectivity prior to any otherness, but is already the result of the subjectivity bestowed by the traversing of the other. Our daily experience, as in the examples given in the previous chapters, shows us how problematic it is to assume that we have or can have a transparent relationship with our own body. When confronted with the fact that not even 'our' images are own, the problem complicates further.

The selfie as an agency

The idea that the selfie represents my 'own' self is what invites Murolo to assume that the selfie allows us to glimpse that it is "from the agency and creativity of social subjects where narratives of oneself are produced that are translated into media formats and genres in order to express ourselves as historical subjects" (Murolo, 2019, p. 119). Instead of staying with Murolo's idea that the use of the selfie is an expression of creativity that evidences the voluntariness and intentionality of the 'social subject,' we should realize that what one could have 'agency' of is the way in which the other has *already* sanctioned and qualified me. The agency over my/self does not come from my simple desire, but from a desire that is already in dialectic with the desire of the other.

We come across this idea of 'agency' very often when talking about how individuals who have been discriminated against in the public space use digital tools, and it is even embarrassing, not to say somewhat condescending and paternalistic, that scholars frequently fall in the trap that, for example, because a transsexual person uses Facebook and takes selfies, then this already makes her selfies a practice of 'greater freedom' or pseudo-subversion. This is how such an act is described by Ana Gutiérrez Martínez (2020, p. 87) when she talks about how a transsexual person and her friends upload selfies on their social networks as a "testimony to the freedom they have taken to inhabit the world as trans feminine people," which challenges the approaches to selfies as "narcissistic and superficial" expressions. However, Gutiérrez never explains how and why those selfies are not narcissistic and superficial; that is, she never explains why a transgender person cannot also be narcissistic and superficial, in line with a simplistic logic that, for the simple fact that she is a trans person, *therefore* her selfies are 'free' of any superficiality, they are 'subverting' social media.

The problem with believing that the *selfie* is a spontaneous presentation of me is that it hides the conditions that overdetermine my/self—that is, that the other has *already* set conditions for me to assume that something is *about* me. This is something never acknowledged by mainstream discourses on 'media literacy,' 'identity appropriation' or 'self-representation': the above-mentioned Murolo (in 2019, p. 120) falls into this error, common in communication and media studies, of believing that because a person frequently uses a tool (like a selfie stick and social media accounts), then one has 'learned' and is 'competent' in its consumption and production, as if the logics of digital image creation and circulation are as simple or clearly executable as those of beating eggs or hammering nails. Communication and media studies, much more often that they openly accept, lose sight of the fact that we should be skeptical of discourse from and about the self, as if only because a person talks about her/himself, especially if that person comes (or we assume that he/she is) from a 'vulnerable group,' then there is no room for discussion or skepticism; there is no room to question agency.

The selfie as a hoax

Evidence that the *selfie* is in no way an expression of 'freedom' or personal identity is that its own digital materiality carries the conditions of possibility to be a constant threat against the subject who creates it. The phenomenon of revenge porn works precisely on this condition: while one way to approach the selfie is as an expression of 'celebration' of one's own body, revenge porn is an expression of punishment towards my own body.

In revenge porn, a person uses the photos or videos they received from another person when they were in some kind of relationship (from flirting or sexting to a committed romantic relationship) to sell them or simply publish them in order to cause embarrassment, blackmail or even physical violence. This supposes the circulation of pornographic material to which the protagonist did not voluntarily agree, and in many cases was not even warned or threatened about beforehand.

The naive thing here would be to reduce the complexity of the issue by saying that revenge porn is an immoral and violent act alien to the nature of the selfie; that is, to assume that the problem is not the selfie but the one who distributes it without consent. But this is where we find that the conditions of the selfie itself only show that the circulation of our own image is something uncontrollable; in fact, it is considered something inherent to the nature of the selfie itself: on one occasion, I heard someone who was afraid of losing his phone because of the pornographic photos he had sent and had been sent. The issue of revenge porn is not exhausted in pointing out the violence of the person who executes it, but in locating the ways in which the digital image, when created by the subject, gives a false sense of ownership over it: the idea that this is *my* image, both as property and for what is shown in it, is precisely the trap of the self the imago supposes. The digital circulation of the selfie in a phenomenon that can be as violent as revenge porn is an extreme that demonstrates the lack of control over images, including those that are 'ours,' and that in less extreme moments this lack of control is noticeable in the fact that the other does not receive our photo as we would like (it is not as applauded with likes or heart emojis as we would like), or possesses our image without our consent (takes pictures of us without our knowledge).

Ayerbe and Cuenca are closer to recognizing how the selfie does not imply a reinforcement of the self that is exhibited in it, but an exhibition of its splitting, of its decentering:

> [T]he identity of the subject of the selfie is never self-centered or given in advance, but always inclined to others and subjected to the affective response of other users of social media. The selfie, ultimately, is not limited to exposing features of a pre-existing identity (although it appears to do just that), but seeks to (self-)define its author within the framework of a "gestural economy of affects."
>
> *(Ayerbe and Cuenca, 2019, p. 5)*

If the *selfie* does not imply the exposure of an already previous identity, but is "always inclined to others and subjected to the affective response of others," we can discard any idea that the selfie is a 'celebration' of 'agency': again, the selfie is not a sample of what 'I already am,' but *a call to the other to recognize what I am.*

To disavow this decentering the selfie imposes on the subject is a trap proper to mainstream communication approaches to the phenomenon that take it as something as obvious as a device that 'communicates' something to others. An example of a very little critical distance to this idea is given by Antonio Fernández Paradas, who even offers us health advice on selfies:

> Someone has commented, quite rightly in some blog, that a healthy person, with a favorable family and personal environment, does not need the compulsive attitude of taking selfies continuously, creating images of himself in order to be accepted by the community […] The healthy attitude would be to take one selfie and enjoy the impact of it on social

media, not to take too many selfies of us so we can have many "likes," which is an addictive attitude, inversely proportional to our self-esteem.
(Fernández Paradas, 2016, pp. 712–713)

We note here one of those attempts of communication studies, so dangerous and naive, to place a kind of psychologized measuring stick: as if there were a clear boundary of how many selfies are already *too many*, as if there was a moment in which our hobby becomes an "addictive attitude," and as if the conditions of production and distribution of these contents were not aimed at always placing us in an "addictive attitude" or redefining the parameters of the same. This imposition of a measuring stick is the correlate of the hypermedicalization of everyday life: of attempts to define what is normal and abnormal, what is too much and too little, the correct ways of relating to each other and living together. Curiously, Fernández never explains to us why "the healthy attitude" would not be simply not to take any selfie, or what to do if it has no impact on social media that I can "enjoy" because nobody cared about my selfie, or if making use of techniques to disguise fatness or ugliness in only one selfie are also part of a "healthy attitude."

How do we establish the threshold from a "healthy attitude" to an "addictive attitude"? We can venture to answer: it depends on how useful the selfie can as an engine of neoliberal production.

The selfie as a neoliberal weapon

Fortunately, there are positions that are critical of the phenomenon, such as that of Estela Roselló Soberón (2018), who elaborates very interesting ethnographic chronicles of social events of the wealthy classes in Mexico City in which the selfie, among other practices, functions to perpetuate conditions of the exhibition, and permanence, of social class status. As I have been mentioning, the selfie cannot be studied as a spontaneous practice or alien to certain interests of production and distribution that, in contemporary life, are the result and perpetuation of a neoliberal subjectivity: the selfie is a sort of right hand of the self-help discourses that pretend to isolate the actions of the subject from the conditions that produce them, so that everyone is 'master of his or her destiny.' Neoliberalism cannot be reduced to a simple economic policy, but it must be verified how it infects human subjectivity to the point of altering even the nature of its happiness: "for the liberal and capitalist mentality and tradition, unhappiness is a factor that affects progress and economic development not only of individuals, but also of nations" (Roselló, 2018, p. 4).

This neoliberal subjectivity is the one that completely erases any boundary between "self-promotion" and "self-exploitation," between a "healthy attitude" and an "addictive attitude": the crossover between one and the other is established by whether it continues to perpetuate conditions and imposition on the subject to exploit itself, in a way that self-exploitation is always through self-promotion.

In this same line, Gabriela Bard and Mariana Magallanes (2021) locate the selfie as a face of the "entrepreneuralization" of the individual. The authors interviewed young people about how they used selfies on Instagram, and noted that even those who do not have a personal 'entrepreneurship' project recognize the logic that social media, subtly or explicitly, imposes on its users to become exploiters of their own image:

> In these contexts, people act as small businesses, watching themselves to accumulate profits that translate into *likes* or followers, guided by the values that circulate within and outside social media. Even those who said in the interviews conducted that they are not interested in collecting followers on Instagram, demonstrate knowledge of the logic of operation on when it is convenient to upload a photo or to post something, how to show oneself, etc. In order to be looked at, it is necessary to understand the forms of regulation of time and the valuable image produced by the capitalist social order.
>
> *(Bard and Magallanes, 2021, p. 7)*

The selfie has thus become, these authors point out, a strategic place for the construction of a commodification of private life: "The emotional sphere has been colonized through the direct commodification of bonds and relationships of care, as well as through the use of emotions as just another commodity" (Bard and Magallanes, 2021, p. 8). The selfie has turned the expression of emotions into a saleable commodity, so that it has managed to phagocytize, under the imperative of exploitation, a tricky feeling of personal freedom. One exposes one's selfie believing that it is a "testimony of freedom," but one can do that only under the condition that, precisely by doing it on digital social media (which is not a public space but a private one), this testimony can be commodified: it is a testimony of the freedom to sell my/self. The authors qualify the use of the selfie in the logic of Instagram as a pedagogy:

> Therefore, [Instagram] serves as a pedagogy of what happiness is, and this responds to "objective" factors that are considered independent of social, historical, political conditioning, that [happiness] would respond to one's own merit and effort. In effect, it reinforces the liberal thought that one can be the architect of one's own life, paradoxical from the moment in which one needs the book written by another person.
>
> *(Bard and Magallanes, 2021, p. 26)*

And this brings us back to Yehya: the conclusion he has on the topic is that "the selfie is a strange expression of honesty but, at the same time, it is the snapshot of a performance, an idealized autobiographical projection in a glimpse of what we would like to be at that precise moment" (Yehya, 2013, p. 283). The selfie is, then, not so much an exhibition of what we are as an exhibition of what we would like to be; that is, the selfie presents the illusion of simply being an exhibition of me, when in fact, as an exhibition of me, it is already *an appeal to the other*, as a request for the other to sanction the image of what we would like to be.

And this brings us back to Burnham too: if the selfie is an appeal to the other, the other side of the coin is the narcissistic, autistic even, solitude the selfie denotes, in the funding characteristics we ascribe them, as a picture taken by the person appearing in them. This means the selfie is a solitude event, even of a "pathetic solitude [...] the selfie denotes a lack of the social" (Burnham, 2018, p. 201). And this even occurs in group selfies, as if the group is a gregarian mass closed to otherness as well.

Instead of showing a spontaneous 'appropriation' of the subject to exposes its 'own' identity, the selfie shows how imprisoned the subject is in its alienation from the other. It is no longer only a matter of locating how the image of the self is being offered for the other, but of realizing that the self, prior to that offering, has no image of its own that is not *already* in relation to the other. The function of the imago offered and assumed in the mirror stage is to insert "a principle of false mastery and fundamental alienation into a synthesis" (Lacan, 1966, p. 566); that is to say, the main function of the self as an imago for the ego is to reinforce the ego by synthesizing it, to subordinate it to an image offered by/to the other, to offer a false mastery of itself, to deceive it into believing that this is its 'own' image.

The reinforcement of our ego through a reinforcement of our self is to deepen in the alienation offered by the imago, to deepen into believing that we are digging into our 'being' to find our 'authentic self' or our 'essence,' yet we actually run into a trap offered by the other. Beyond our selfie, in the depths of ourselves, we can only find the other.

Notes

1 An idea presented in various Freudian texts is that language and speech are the seeds for human civilization and culture for they are substitutes of actions, and that, as far as we know, animals don't have such devices. To this idea, we find a phrase that is popularly, and mistakenly, attributed to Freud, who refers to it in an early text (from 1893): "the man who first flung a word of abuse at his enemy instead of a spear was the founder of civilization" (Freud, 1962/III, p. 36).

2 Freud says, in *Civilization and Its Discontents* (1961/XXI, p. 111), that the other is "someone who tempts them to satisfy their aggressiveness on him."

3 My examples come from Mexico and Latin America; I am sure that this problem, with some nuances, is present in academia all over the world.

4 That is to say, while a somewhat naïve position would believe that technology is the result of certain subjectivities, we must rather recognize that technology is *the producer of certain subjectivities.*

References

Ayerbe, Nerea & Cuenca, Jaime. (2019). "El selfie como performance de la identidad. Explorando la performatividad de la auto-imagen desde el arte de acción." *Papeles del CEIC*, Vol. 2019, No. 2, pp. 1–16.

Bard Wigdor, Gabriela & Magallanes Udovicich, Mariana Loreta. (2021). "Instagram: la búsqueda de la felicidad desde la autopromoción de la imagen." *Revista Culturales*, Vol. 9, No. 1, 29 pgs.

Burnham, Clint. (2018). "Lacan and New Media." In Ankhi Mukherjee (editor). *After Lacan. Literature, Theory, and Psychoanalysis in the Twenty-First Century.* Cambridge University Press, pp. 185–205.

Fernández Paradas, Antonio Rafael. (2016). "La mercantilización del selfie como medio de construcción de las identidades sociales." *Opción*, Vol. 32, No. 9, pp. 706–717.

Freud, Sigmund. [1893] (1962). "On The Psychical Mechanism of Hysterical Phenomena: A Lecture." In *The Standard Edition of The Complete Psychological Works of Sigmund Freud*, Vol. III. The Hogarth Press, pp. 24–39.

Freud, Sigmund. [1895] (1966). "Project For a Scientific Psychology." In *The Standard Edition of The Complete Psychological Works of Sigmund Freud*, Vol. I. The Hogarth Press, pp. 281–397.

Freud, Sigmund. [1930] (1961). "Civilization and Its Discontents." In *The Standard Edition of The Complete Psychological Works of Sigmund Freud*, Vol. XXI. The Hogarth Press, pp. 57–145.

Gutiérrez Martínez, Ana Paulina. (2020). "Cambios y permanencias en la atmósfera cultural trans femenina de la Ciudad de México." *Estudios Sociológicos de El Colegio de México*, Vol. 38, No. 112, pp. 73–102.

Lacan, Jacques. [1948] (2006). "Aggressiveness in Psychoanalysis." In *Écrits. The First Complete Edition in English.* W.W. Norton & Company, pp. 82–101.

Lacan, Jacques. [1949] (2006). "The Mirror Stage as Formative of the *I* Function as Revealed in Psychoanalytic Experience." In *Écrits. The First Complete Edition in English.* W.W. Norton & Company, pp. 75–81.

Lacan, Jacques. [1960] (2006). "Remarks on Daniel Lagache's Presentation: 'Psychoanalysis and Personality Structure'." In *Écrits. The First Complete Edition in English.* W.W. Norton & Company, pp. 543–574.

Murolo, Norberto Leonardo. (2015). "Del mito del Narciso a la *selfie.* Una arqueología de los cuerpos codificados." *Palabra Clave*, Vol. 18, No. 3, pp. 676–700.

Murolo, Norberto Leonardo. (2019). "Teoría de la selfi. Narrativa y usos de la fotografía digital contemporánea." In *deSignis*, Vol. 30, No. 19, pp. 115–122.

Roselló Soberón, Estela. (2018). "*Happiness made in Mexico*: lujo, consumo y felicidad entre las clases medias altas de las Lomas de Chapultepec (Ciudad de México, 2018)." *Relaciones. Estudios de Historia y Sociedad*, Vol. 41, No. 163, pp. 1–33.

Yehya, Naief. (2013). *Pornocultura: el espectro de la violencia sexualizada en los medios.* Tusquets.

6

PSYCHOLOGIST BARBIE AND WORKER KEN

The Traps of the Self

Communication and desire (of the other)

Moving away from the idea of an *already* formed ego, becoming aware of the intrusion of the subject as a residue that prevents the fortification of the ego, locating the other as fundamental to the constitution of the ego, we now come across one of Lacan's most famous aphorisms, reformulated several times through his teaching, which introduces us to the third consequence of the mirror stage: the desire of the subject is the desire of the other. In the text on aggressiveness, Lacan says: "[the ego] this form crystallizes in the subject's inner conflictual tension, which leads to the awakening of his desire for the object of the other's desire" (1966, p. 92). What does it mean that *the desire of the ego is the desire for the object of the other's desire*?

The way it is formulated in the previous quotation, the formula allows for two readings:

1. *to desire the object that the other desires*: we have seen this in relation to the birth of one's own subjectivity through jealousy and family relationships, and we recognize it very frequently in young infants, who begin to be interested in an object or toy that they had been ignoring until someone else takes it;
2. *to desire to be the object of the other's desire*: this refers to wanting to take the place of the other's object of desire, to become the object that the other desires. This is the interpretation we will focus on in this section, as it is the most important point, at this stage of Lacanian thought, in which we highlight the "dialectic of identifications" (Lacan, 1966, p. 91), in which the subject introjects the other's desire, identifies with that desire.

DOI: 10.4324/9781003640653-6

Either of these two readings allows us to recognize that the ego assumes as its own objects of desire those that are objects of desire of the other: from a toy to the identity of selfhood offered by the other. Even in desire, that inner and subjective force that one would believe—outside the psychoanalytic realm—to be spontaneous and personal, we can locate the figure of the other as an axis that does not allow us to assume the existence of an inner or authentic subject.

Let's go back Seminar 1, in continuation with the previous quote on the body of the subject:

> It is within the see-saw movement, the movement of exchange with the other, that man becomes aware of himself as body, as the empty form of the body. In the same way, everything which is then within him in a pure state of desire, original desire, unconstituted and confused, which finds expression in the wailing of the child—he will learn to recognise it through its inversion in the other. He will learn, because he has not yet learned, in as much as we have not brought communication into play.
>
> *(Lacan, [1954] 1988, p. 170)*

This quote offers us nothing less than a first Lacanian definition of communication[1]: *the process in which we learn to adopt the desire of the other as our own desire*, the recognition *in our own* inner desire of something that is *in the other.* In this idea, we can understand why Lacan, interested in the Imaginary, is so interested in identification: it is through identification that the ego appropriates something that is other, that erases the boundary between the interior and the exterior. Communication is a way to produce and mask the transversal function the other has in the constitution of the ego.

Freud noted (1966/I, p. 331), as we have discussed already, that the other is the first object towards which we have *both hostile and friendly* impulses, insofar as it is, at the same time, the first object that causes *displeasure and pleasure.* Lacan clearly maintains this position, which functions as a correlate of this idea of communication: the birth of subjectivity supposes identification with the desire of the other.

Against this psychoanalytic approach, the psychologized position operates by offering a discourse that aims to deny the place of the other in the foundation of human subjectivity. The advantage of this position is that it can offer an account of the social bond (and the problems of the social bond) from the presumption of an ego that exists and that relates to other egos that, beyond the relationship they have with each other, have certain characteristics of their own and with which that relationship begins to be constructed. In other words, for the psychologization that aims to strengthen the sense of self to please the ego, the ego exists, has a sense of self, and then it is this *whole self* that builds bonds with other selves. Psychologized communication is that of a complete self with another complete self. The criticism of communication made by psychoanalysis is that the self this psychologized approach presumes has already incorporated the desire of the other as a condition of possibility to affirm its completeness.

From an attempt to dethrone the empire of the ego, of a logic that goes against reinforcing the ego, psychoanalysis asks about *the other within the ego*: it is not that first there is an ego and then comes the bond with the other, but that the bond with the other and the birth of the ego are part of the same act, like that famous drawing by M. C. Escher of hands painting themselves (*Drawing Hands*, 1948).

As a matter of fact, we can say that psychoanalysis is more radical than only affirming this, for it is a project that sustains itself by *operating directly against the ego*, since the first resistance to analysis is the ego itself: "the ego represents the center of all resistances to the treatment of symptoms" (Lacan, 1966, p. 96). As clinical experience shows us, whether as analysts or analysands, the first thing that operates to avoid the continuation of the analysis are the symptoms of the ego that is attacked by the analytic device.

What are the consequences of this difference between psychoanalysis and psychologizing practices? Why does psychoanalysis warn of a certain skepticism against the reinforcement of the ego? The reinforcement of the ego that some psychological practices, economic systems and political discourses celebrate today, in the neoliberalism of identities, in the market of the selves, are consistent, totalized, objectified *images of the self*: multiple identity options from which one, freely (so they tell us), chooses.

The sovereign self (and its identity politics)

In her very deep and controversial essay on this topic, Elisabeth Roudinesco (2022) characterizes our current era as one of a popularization, in public discourse, of what she calls *a sovereign self*, a "self-affirmation—transformed into self-inflation—[which] would thus be the distinctive sign of an epoch in which each individual seeks to be himself or herself as sovereign, as king or queen rather than as someone else" (pp. xi–x). There is no space for encounter, confrontation, dialectic or understanding of otherness in the times of a sovereign self, but only a 'celebration of the self' that goes through its reductionism and the establishment of hierarchies, even in hierarchies of suffering and victimhood.

Roudinesco's text goes through a discussion of the ways in which categories such as gender (as opposed to sex), racialization (as opposed to racism), the postcolonial (as opposed to the critique of the colonial) and identity replacement (as opposed to the critique of systems of exploitation) are occupying places in the public discussion, and tend to become banners that 'left-wing' movements and groups (whether they call themselves that or are called that by others) raise in a rather superficial and caricatured defense of deeper discussions that took place before their existence (and even parallel to them). Roudinesco argues, especially in the penultimate chapter of her book, that these 'left-wing' movements, popularly grouped as the 'woke' movement, uphold the same perverse logics that work in the conspiracy theories of the ultra-right and the alt-right that elevate figures such as Donald Trump and Elon Musk[2]:

> Nothing is more regressive for civilization and socialization than to align oneself with a hierarchy of identities and memberships. To be sure, the assertion of an identity is always an attempt to counter the erasure of oppressed minorities, but it proceeds through an excess of self-centered claims, or even through a mad desire not to mix with any community but one's own.
>
> *(Roudinesco, 2022, p. 6)*

The world of the sovereign self is one of the hierarchization of individuality and the expulsion of otherness: we would not understand the concept of "*safe space*," as it is practiced in many public places, if it were not for the popularity of these logics. The sovereign self is a world of continuous *segregation* of the self, separation from the other: the separation from the other sustained in a "self-enclosure of self-identified victims" (p. 85).

Roudinesco does not use such a word, but we can definitely ascribe the discourses she criticizes as examples of 'woke' or SJW (*social justice warrior*) logic: an attempt to fight against the social, structural and historical injustices that exist even in countries that in the West would be considered the least unequal. What Roudinesco criticizes is not, of course, the fight against, for example, the gender pay gap, but rather the fact that the logic of such a fight is rooted in a celebration of the self, in the presumption that identity is a process that begins and ends with the individual who speaks of him/herself (i.e., his/her self), and that sustains his identity on an exclusion (more or less implicit) of otherness. This is the foundation of liberal identity politics, which began to dominate public discussions in the West after the fall of the USSR, using the USA as its most popular platform: "commitment to identity politics took the place of classic militancy, especially at the heart of the American left" (Roudinesco, 2022, p. 13).

Many of us watched with sad laughter when fashion magazines, which have sustained themselves for decades by using women's bodies as mannequins that establish the conditions of Western beauty, called themselves 'allies' of women who were harassed by Hollywood producers; however, for some it might be an additional surprise that psychiatry and psychology are important participants in this logic, as accomplices in the hyperpathologization of life that exalts the sovereign self. That is how manuals like the famous DSM (*Diagnostic and Statistical Manual for Mental Disorders*), by the American Psychiatric Association, work on patients: they set aside conceptual elaborations from psychoanalysis and classical psychiatry to embrace cognitivism, behaviorism and neurosciences, in alliance with the pharmaceutical industries which, without hesitation, celebrate the idea of having more diseases to diagnose:

> In other words, instead of defining the human subject according to a tripartite social, biological, and psychological approach, this new psychiatry retained just one component, behavior, or rather "behavioral difference," set up as an infinitely extendable system: the focus was no longer on subjective units but rather on identitarian variations according to each behavior.
>
> *(Roudinesco, 2022, pp. 21–22)*

These "identitarian variations" are what sustain a model that diagnoses depression according to a chronological temporality fixed in advance, not according to the way in which each subject expresses its depressive state. It was these "identitarian variations" that produced, as Roudinesco explains later in the book (p. 106), a proliferation of phobias in the DSM that were exported from/to identity struggles: homophobia, transphobia, fatphobia, and a long etcetera. The problem was not, it must be emphasized, the fight against discrimination against homosexuals; the problem is that, being based on a behaviorist, cognitivist and hyperbiologized understanding of the human subject, these identity struggles ended up *pathologizing discrimination*: as we often see in the most absurd psychologizing interpretations, for example, when indicating that acts of discriminatory violence are a developmental disorder (or of 'attachment,' or of lack of 'emotional regulation,' to mention other psychologizing mantras[3]). We are not only discriminating against some people when we say 'hate speech,' but we actually discriminate because we are mentally ill.

These *identitarian variations*, certainly indicative of an *identitarian drift* (as the subtitle of the original title of Roudinesco's book suggests), are indicative of a model of society that only admits diversity, but not difference. What does this mean?

When we talk about *identity politics*, along Roudinesco's lines of thought, we talk about politics recognize in the identity of the sovereign self the place from which the political struggle is established, i.e., the political struggle is fought within the realm of the self. The difference between the identity politics of the far right and that of the liberal 'left' is based on how they relate to identity diversity: the far right cannot deal with identity diversity, the liberal 'left' embraces identity diversity. For example, before the legalization of same-sex marriage, or at least, if not total legalization, its open discussion, 'heteronormative' identity was *the identity* (more specifically, it was the *only* identity considered the '*normal*' sexual identity). Opposed to heteronormative identity, every other sexual identity was considered a perverse or immoral act, a *deviant identity*. This is still true among the far right (and, more implicitly, in the alt-right). As the participation of the homosexual community in public life became more visible decades ago, even up to the legal acceptance of marriage, that identity that was previously *deviant* is now accepted as *another identity*, which jeopardizes the place of 'normal identity' that was previously the heteronormative identity; that is, the acceptance of a 'deviant' identity as an accepted one destroys the place of exception of the 'normal' identity. Against this logic, liberal identity politics has managed to create a politics of identity diversity, into which there are many identities accepted within the realm of the public.

Now, there is a catch in this acceptance, besides the problem of how this acceptance seems to be done under the condition of pathologizing those who do not accept, as was mentioned some paragraphs ago. There is an even more structural problem in this, which points us to the need to distinguish between *diversity and difference*. Let's consider the following example from my personal experience. At a talk on indigenous cinema, the speaker, an indigenous filmmaker, spoke of the different practices of learning, pre-production, filming, post-production and distribution of films in and from her own territorial community. At one point in the presentation, she indicated that the development of her scripts and stories was aimed at "preserving the traditions" of her community. During the Q&A time, a woman in the audience took the microphone and said that she is also an indigenous person (although a different community than the speaker), and pointed out that she has no interest in preserving the traditions of her place of origin, traditions with which she does not identify and which have caused her and her family so much damage. Read from the perspective of diversity, what we would note here are two life experiences that propose two different ways of understanding (or assuming) indigenous identity. The problem with this position is that it falls into the idea that there are two ways of *indigenousness* that can coexist, and that both positions are 'valid,' even though the second might be more uncomfortable: such is the *diversity of identities* that there is not *only one* way to be indigenous, there are *multiple* indigenous identities, and so on. However, the second intervention doesn't simply present *another* identity position, but *a conflict within identity itself*: there is no way to escape the conflict when we read it from the perspective of *identity difference*; that is, this tension makes it clear to us that being indigenous is not about 'preserving traditions' or 'doing away with traditions,' but rather the very conflict that exists between what is preserved and what is destroyed in traditions.

In other words, the politics of identity *diversity* understand identity as *something*—that is, as something that possesses certain characteristics, more or less recognizable or assumable. Identity as something in the order of diversity bets on a *segregation*, the main feature of what Roudinesco calls an *identitarian drift* (2022, p. 77), a phenomenon present in discourses from *both* ultraracist groups and political correctness collectives.

Identity politics are the politics of diversity. What does a politics of *difference* look like?

The politics of difference only recognizes identity in a point that *disturbs* the constitution of a totalizing identity: difference is not the difference between one and the other (that is a matter of diversity), but of conflict immanent to the establishment of that very diversity. It is hard for me to give an example that doesn't come from a local perspective, but that's precisely my point: only from within the 'identity' can I find the problem of identity. Mexicans who read this might agree that the issue with the *quesadilla* is a particular good example. Where is 'Mexican identity' to be found? It is not to be found in those objects or images that come to mind when we read 'Mexican identity,' but in the places that are conflictive *only for Mexicans*: Mexicans define themselves by that which disturbs the completeness of *Mexicanness.* The quesadilla is a trademark of Mexican cuisine, and a discussion within the country is if it *must* have cheese (most of Mexico thinks that way), or if it could not have it and *still* be called quesadilla (something that happens only in Mexico City and the regions adjacent to it). This might seem to be a banal thing, but the only country where the nature of the quesadilla is a topic of hot discussion, sometimes more and sometimes less subtly hostile, is Mexico. And it is precisely this point of conflict where *the difference in identity* that inhabits the interior of 'Mexicanness' is recognized: what is Mexican is not a dish, nor is a 'true' quesadilla the emblem of 'true' Mexicanness, but the *conflict itself* about whether or not *this* quesadilla is a *truly Mexican* dish.[4]

The politics of identitarian diversity are committed to a harmonious coexistence between identities: regardless of our racial identity, gender identity, ethnic identity (among many others), we can find the conditions to live in a harmonious, equal, 'safe' way. There is, however, an impasse in this logic, for there is an identity that *cannot* be understood in diversity: class identity. While the discourses that advocate for identitarian diversity seek the conditions of equilibrium between a diversity of identities, class identity is presented as the abject, the symptom of the bond in diversity. While we can imagine relationships of total parity between diverse identities, it is impossible to imagine a relationship of parity between capitalists and workers, since, by definition, one finds oneself in the position of exploiting the other.

This impossibility of conceiving a relationship of equals between capitalists and workers is the reason why class identity is presented, in Marxism, as an identity crossed by its incapacity for completeness, as an identity that is divided in itself: it is a non-totalizing identity. This is why class politics do not function in the same dimension as the politics of identity recognition, because *the class difference* is precisely what the *class struggle* aims to abolish. The class struggle, as Žižek indicates (2018, p. 127), is not simply *another* antagonism that is placed on the list of antagonisms (racial, sexual, ethnic), but is, in capitalism, the very *overdetermination* of those antagonisms. That is why the class struggle is on the side of *difference itself*, because its resolution does not bet on a just coexistence between diverse classes: the only solution to the class struggle is the abolition of all classes. It is because of this fundamental question that in 'dialogues' such as those in which businessmen and union leaders meet with members of parliament, in governments trapped in global neoliberalism, even those who claim to be left-wing (like most Western 'liberal' democracies), it is naive to pretend that there is a level playing field in this dialogue: it is ridiculous or perverse that when the proletariat, for example, asks for a reduction in working hours, this is equated with employers asking for no reduction because it lowers their prospects for 'productivity.' It is impossible to say that it is the same thing when a worker asks to work fewer hours or when an employer asks to earn the same money as the hours they will no longer pay: there is no balance in 1 coin more to the worker than 1 coin less to the employer. Equal quantity of money is not equality in class struggle: this is why it is *impossible* to include class struggle as an identity struggle. When we notice the celebration that neoliberalism makes of identity politics, we should verify that this commitment to diversity has the effect of canceling out any truly emancipatory politics, insofar as it is a commitment to diversity *under market conditions.* Thus, we can understand neoliberalism as *a free market of identities.*

This distinction between diversity and difference jeopardizes theoretical and political projects such as *intersectionality.* In an article dedicated to criticizing the most naive approaches to this concept, David Pavón-Cuéllar and María Concepción Lizeth Capulín Arellano (2023, p. 71) comment that intersectional approaches fail to escape an imaginary logic of identity, under the pretense of a sovereign self: intersectionality is not only not radical but rather dull in its possibilities, as it never questions or doubts individual experience or the desire that feeds the subject's conscience: the basis of intersectionality is that the individual experience of the suffering subject is never questioned, as intersectionality itself is an individual masquerade of a more fundamental structure of exploitation (colonial and heteropatriarchal). Intersectionality divides and categorizes discourses that oppress the subject, and does not conceive of the way in which the subject itself crosses these categories: it confuses causes with consequences (p. 72).

> This is why psychoanalysis and Marxism (when they are truly radical) are discourses that are difficult to understand from intersectional approaches, as they call into question individual experience, the discourse of consciousness and imaginary relationships; not simply to say that these are expressions of something 'false,' but to go *across* them in order to understand how the subject weakens the structures that try to reduce subjectivity to predisposed categories, even those that explain suffering and exploitation. Intersectionality has become a powerful ally to depoliticize and psychologize subjective experiences, confining the individual to "a primarily individual, psychological, and only secondarily collective, political sphere. In this sphere, there is an irresistible tendency

> to depoliticization and psychologization, dissolving the structure into what is experienced intersectionally by each individual."
>
> *(Pavón-Cuéllar & Capulín Arellano, 2023, p. 74)*

This may explain, among other things, why the global left has abandoned a universal and collective vocation to focus on the defense of particular identities: by reducing political experience and emancipation to what *each individual* aims to achieve, ending up psychologizing politics and depoliticizing the psyche. This produces an atomization of individual experience not unrelated to a logic of hyperindividualization of the experience… of consumption. Neoliberalism is built on the pretense of sustaining this ultra-individual experience, and this is evident in the construction of algorithms for advertisements on digital social media: *it is individual advertising*, and therefore it is advertising that sustains the empire of egoic individuality.

Back to Roudinesco. This experience of the celebration of individuality, which is the support of the explosion of a free market of identities, coincided with the end of the Cold War and the establishment of a (supposedly) unipolar world where liberal capitalist democracy reigns. As the years went by and the capitalism established in the countries that used to conform the Soviet Union did not provide better conditions than before for all citizens, and neoliberalism finished off (not only *the Left* but) what was left of the welfare state in the West, an eternal "exaltation of the self" was established, exalted in the idea of 'happiness' that neoliberalism sells:

> In this respect, in the Western world, the immense expansion of therapies offering happiness, coaching, personal development, meditation therapies, resilience institutes, and other groups focused on exalting or repairing the self, allied with the growing consumption of psychotropic drugs well beyond the classic psychiatric prescriptions—all this is the sign of a social inability to face up to the question of happiness, a collective and individual ideal, as it had been conceptualized by the Enlightenment thinkers and their heirs.
>
> *(Roudinesco, 2022, p. 140)*

The problem with the identitarian diversity politics of the liberal 'left' is that the price paid for the victories in favor of historically attacked identities has been to believe that the recognition of identity can only be achieved through a celebration of the empire of the self. This celebration is very functional to the neoliberal market, as it helps to sustain it: certainly, neoliberalism has a much broader perspective of identity diversity than the ecclesiastical, conservative or autocratic elites, but it has this broader perspective not out of altruistic disinterest, but because the essential thing is to achieve *the hypercategorization of identity*, to make identity quantifiable, measurable, objectifiable, managing to create an illusion of openness to identities that is actually an openness "dominated as it is by objectifying ends" (Lacan, 1966, p. 96). Identity politics in neoliberalism only understand the potential of each identity insofar as each self is its own 'niche market.'

The spectacular self (in its stupidest reality)

Probably the most classic and pertinent place for this discussion is Guy Debord's T*he Society of the Spectacle* of 1967 (1995). The point of the society of the spectacle is that the illusion of equality can only coexist in the empire of separation: the spectacle is an instrument that creates an illusion of unification via separation. The logic of the spectacle is not that of a simple decoration or supplement to a world that is 'real,' but rather that it "is both the outcome and the goal of the dominant mode of production" (Debord, 1995, p. 13, § 6). What does this mean?

In a world where identity is expressed, and strengthened, through images that function as imagos for the subject, the symptomatic thing to identify is the way in which that image is constructed as imago. If the very imago of the self is neither spontaneous nor natural, nor is alien to the intervention of the other, we must also realize that the mechanisms for sustaining this imago are not naive or innocent in sustaining the empire of the self. Thus, we verified in a previous chapter that the places where the selfie is presented are not simply the places of exhibition of the selfie but also are the conditions and logics of creation (i.e., a selfie is only a selfie insofar it is distributed in social media). That is the point of Debord's concept of the *spectacle of* society: the spectacle is not simply the product of the spectacle (the mass media products being the most obvious instances), but *the conditions for the spectacle to continue to be maintained*, for spectacle is both the product and the producer; the consumption of the spectacle is at the same time the production of the spectacle.[5]

In a world governed by this logic of the spectacle, we notice the intensity with which we are pushed, to show 'our' identity, to be who we 'really' are, without any concealment. The problem is not that I decide to be in this or that way; the problem is a certain naivety in believing that our identity is spontaneous, *our own*, without having been previously sanctioned by the other, already offered to the other, and that we can only have this or that identity if it is being shown as 'our true' identity.

The current era is reminiscent of a commercial that aired in Mexico (I'm sure there was a similar campaign in many countries) in the early 2000s for a new line of Barbie dolls, whose slogan was "I am what I want to be, I am a Barbie girl," while gymnast Barbies, model Barbies, chef Barbies and others are presented on screen: to what extent does 'our' identity not respond to one of the offers on the market of identities? How 'spontaneous' or 'ours' is the decision we make if the options to choose from have already been sanctioned, verified, approved by the other? Let's not be mistaken, these identity options are not simply the result of socio-historical changes in society: if the market offers those identities to us, it is because they are ways of *objectifying our subjectivities*, of reducing us to the gymnast, the model, the chef or the Barbie of fashion, because all the diversity of professions does not matter *as long as we are Barbies*. The essential thing is that we believe that these decisions are 'free' of any influence from the other, so, in a way, *Barbie is a Lacanian mechanism of communication*: it allows me to assume as *my* desire whatever is the object of desire of the other, it allows me to mask the way the desire of the other constitutes my/self, or as Roudinesco sentences in the aforementioned text: each one "became themselves through crossdressing" (2022, p. 15)—that is, I can only become my/self by transforming into another.[6]

This is something never addressed in the naive representation of the problem of identity presented in the film *Barbie* (dir. Greta Gerwig, 2023), which reaches the absurd paroxysm that the 'authentic' identity of myself as a Barbie is when another Barbie points out a 'contradiction' in my behavior; I'm talking about the scene in which the Barbies 'wake up' from their patriarchal hypnosis thanks to another Barbie telling them the 'contradictions' of life as a woman. The grotesque ingenuity of this is in the fact that the contradiction is not appropriated, questioned or rejected: the contradiction is pointed out in order to annul its role in the constitution of identity, so that, and *by doing away with the contradiction*, I can *regain a* 'complete' identity. Thus, in *Barbie*, identity is complete: contradiction doesn't destabilize or deconstruct identity; it is, on the contrary, the precise thing that allows me to achieve a full identity. Contradiction in identity is useful insofar it erects the phallus of the self-identity (remember the Barbie doll in the first scene of the film).

A much more complex and interesting film that received much less attention and discussion than Gerwig's childish movie is *Women Talking* (dir. Sarah Polley, 2022). In the film, a group of women from a Mennonite community who discover they have been systematically drugged and raped by men in their group meet up to discuss how to resolve the vote (only among the women) that was tied between staying to fight the men or fleeing. In the title alone, we can see the enormous difference in how they understand femininity: while *Barbie* is the embodiment of *an* ideal of the phallic self, *Women Talking* is about *several* women who are *talking*, discussing, dialoguing, sometimes with laughter and sometimes with hostility, sometimes in agreement and sometimes in disagreement, with the presence of a man who acts as *an other who challenges*, in a dialectic that one of the characters marvelously sums up: "When we have liberated ourselves, we will have to ask ourselves who we are."

Barbie inhabits the world of psychologized, totalized and totalizing identity where *the other is told who she is*, while *Women Talking* inhabits the world of fragmented identity and dialectical identification, where *a space is opened up for the question of who one is.* An important scene at the beginning of the latter film brings into dialogue this space for questioning that the first film never opens: "'Leaving' and 'fleeing' are different words with different meanings. They each say something about us." Despite the fact that, materially speaking, both events (fleeing and leaving) result in an identical consequence (women are no longer here), the subjective position is highly different, so the consequences might not be so identical: there is no guarantee, there is only a *possibility* to open a question with regard to our own identity. The conflictive and contradictory nature of my identity is at the core of my identity; thus, *Women Talking* proves to be a much more intelligent film to question ourselves than the plain, naive imago *Barbie* offers, which is the precise correlation of the function the Barbie dolls have in the offer of an identity to cling to.

In popular speech, we notice these in the memes with which we 'identify,' in which we say that 'it is literally me': a funny or embarrassing scene that exhibits an excess of subjectivity to which we anchor our/selves. For such things, the Lacan of the 1950s and 1960s, the Lacan of the Imaginary, was concerned with the formation of the ego through identification, and thought that the Freudian text *par excellence* on the topic of identification, *Group Psychology and the Analysis of the Ego*, was so important. See this point in his text on Daniel Lagache's presentation (from 1960):

> For the question he raises in *Group Psychology and the Analysis of the Ego* is how an object, reduced to its stupidest reality, but functioning for a certain number of subjects as a common denominator (confirming what I will say momentarily about its function as an insignia), can bring about an identification of the ideal ego with the very moronic power of misadventure that the ideal ego turns out to be at its core.
>
> *(Lacan, 1966, p. 567)*

Once an object "reduced to its stupidest reality" (i.e., in its simple existence) is established as what defines a community of subjects, they assume that object as an ideal ego with which they identify. What Freud called "mental infection" (1955/XVIII, p. 107) is the fact that a trait not only manages to become the subject's denominator—that is, manages to reduce the subject to *that trait*—but also becomes a common denominator as it manages to enthrone itself as the *identifying trait* of a community of subjects. The identifying mental infection is that one reduces one's singular subjectivity to the same common trait as other subjects, imposing a regime of *false community*, since it is passed off as an individual choice what was an identification with (the desire of) the other; and as the Lacanian quote at the beginning of this chapter would say, this regime of false community is a regime of communication. See this idea in his *The Situation of Psychoanalysis and the Training of Psychoanalysts in 1956*:

> Identification with the image that gives the group its ideal—which is here the image of sufficiency incarnate—certainly founds [...] the communion of the group, but it is precisely at the expense of all articulate communication.
>
> *(Lacan, 1966, p. 410)*

In reference to something similar, Lacan spoke, in an even earlier text—1936's *Beyond the "Reality Principle"*—of an *emotional communication*,

> which is essential to social groups and manifests itself immediately enough in the fact that man exploits his semblable, recognizes himself in this semblable, and is attached to this semblable by the indelible psychical link that perpetuates the truly specific vital misery of his first years of life.
>
> *(1966, p. 70)*

Communication allows the illusion of a libidinously linked community, in order to hide the fact that this community is based on the exploitation of one person by another.

In the world of 'niche market' marketing, Freud's identification as a mental infection operates quite perversely among young people, who take their generation etiquette as "an object, reduced to its stupidest reality": from so-called 'millennials,' 'generation Z,' 'zoomers' or 'boomers,' among many other categories, ignoring the economic and social structures that created these labels, trying to apply them in a context that is alien to the one they had at the time, reducing the cultural and economic differences among them in such grotesque caricature labels as they use them as an excuse or explanation for their attitudes against people of different age, against authority figures or as a justification for their own subjective implications in the problems they claim to suffer. The market has offered them these labels that tell them 'what it's like' to be someone born in a particular year, and they verify that this label is 'correct' in their behavior. The way these empty names work is the same as a horoscope or a fortune cookie; the sad thing is that this logic is what is implemented in the university: those of us who teach know how the educational psychology departments of universities have a special inclination for reducing the complexities of today's youth to this 'sort-of' classificatory system in order to justify not asking students to read because, as I was told at a 'teacher training' session at a 'prestigious' university in Mexico, "Generation Z is more visual."

The object in its most stupid reality into which we anchor our subjectivity is also present in each issue that enters the 'public debate' on the 'emotional' side, as it is common for social media to allow us to *automatically* indicate that we are on one side or another on a conflict, or ascribe under a certain belief or conviction: we see this in pre-programmed banners and filters for profile photos in the month of March (on violence against women), in June (in support of the gender-diverse community), with the flag of a country when it suffers a terrorist attack (of course, French flags in November 2015, Ukrainian flags in February 2022, Israel flags in October 2023, curiously enough, not as easy to program a Palestinian flag). How can we fail to notice that these little flags and colors are a common denominator in which the subject, psychically infected by identification, assumes an ideal ego? Since, in digital social media, it is not a matter of public discussion but a matter of maintaining a coherent, reinforced and simple imago in front of the other, we realize that before having any conviction (or clarifying the conditions and sacrifices of that conviction), it is necessary to *let the other know* that I have the conviction of an ideal self.

This ideal ego, the imago we promote on social media, has created the conditions for very specific characters that could not have been conceived of before its emergence. I am referring here to the figure *par excellence* of the self-exploitation of the digital imago: the *influencer*. As the name suggests, the *influencer* is not simply a figure 'who influences something,' but their role is *influence itself*. The fame they enjoy is comparable to that previously only enjoyed by film and television stars (with the exception that those stars act), and before them by medieval royalty (with the exception that those figures possessed a specific political power). The influencer is just that: a figure who influences; they do not have a specific characteristic of what they are 'influential' in. A definition I heard at a conference about one of these figures, Kim Kardashian, hit the nail accurately: Kim Kardashian is not famous for something she does or did in the past, but she is famous *because* she is Kim Kardashian. This tautology, the absence of any clear commitment on anything beyond the maintaining of her own image, is what explains why there are influencers about everything: food, makeup, politics, travel and, in the most regrettable cases, even philosophy, psychoanalysis and activism. The magical power given to royalty in medieval times is not so different from the power of influencers to, for example, bankrupt a restaurant by reporting mistreatment or discrimination of some kind. It is irrelevant whether or not this mistreatment took place, or the vicissitudes of the situation: the influencer who believes himself to be a kind of pseudo-activist on social media, in reality, only exists on the condition that the promotion he/she does is, above any kind of cause, that of *his/her own image*. The difference between activism that was born before or outside the logic of digital social media and the activism of the influencer is the function of phagocytosis and superordination of the image: digital activism understood from the perspective of influencers on Instagram, X, Facebook and TikTok has the interest, before any feminist, environmentalist, animalist or anti-discrimination cause, of *sustaining the empire of the self*, the empire of the imago, for the other. In a dialectical turn, the 'digital activist influencer' is, first and foremost, an activist for the imago.

The canceling self (and its superego)

The reinforcement of the self of social media activism (commonly found under hashtags such as #IamX, #raiseawereness) is committed to a non-split ego, and, in the end, to establish a very strong superego that functions as a mechanism of eternal hypervigilance based on the digital footprint (as when an actress is 'exposed' in the tweets she posted several years ago) and in placing ourselves before the eyes of others whom we probably don't even know (the 'friends' and 'followers' of the social media accounts). This superego is what operates in the punitive mechanisms of politically correct discourse, which establish a position of judgment that goes well beyond any attempt to denounce an injustice: eternal hypervigilance is necessary over those who are punished. It is not coincidental that Lacan found, in his 1950 text *A Theoretical Introduction to the Functions of Psychoanalysis in Criminology*, obvious connections between the superego and the mechanisms of punishment in contemporary societies, in which it is not enough for someone to be found guilty and punished, but rather a "subjective assent" is required (Lacan, 1966, p. 103) for punishment to really mean something: it is not enough for someone to be punished, but it is required for them to *accept themselves as punished by others*. This is what happens in the episode "White Bear" from the series *Black Mirror* (created by Charlie Brooker, 2011–): a woman complicit in a violent crime against a girl is punished daily in a circus show that is used as a pedagogy of punishment, so that it is not enough to punish her or to know that she is paying for her crime in prison, because today's world of entertainment needs to *see her subjective assent*, in the form of suffering her own punishment. That is the politically correct discourse on which the most naive, punitive and superegoic digital 'activism' is based: taking a sort of enjoyment in the fact that the other is being punished.

Roudinesco hypothesizes that this state of affairs bears a painful relationship to the way in which the humanities and social sciences abandoned Marxist and ideological critique paradigms, and have decanted, in recent decades, into a kind of contest of suffering:

> After 2015, the identitarian evolution of [intersectional] "studies" took a political turn with the appearance of major punitive campaigns orchestrated by groups adopting the classifications developed in the heart of academic institutions. By going out into the streets, these "studies" ended up providing support for what is called cancel culture, another widespread practice on social networks; all this took place against a background of increasing racism, (American) supremacism, and terror of Islamism. This "culture" consists in pointing fingers, for the purpose of ostracism or elimination, at a person, an association, or an institution whose statements, mores, acts, or habits are judged "offensive" toward one minority or another.

> The culture of public denunciation, always dangerous for democracy, whatever its good or bad intentions may be, goes hand in hand with other forms of counterattack, like those targeting "cultural appropriation." […] This is a fascinating Pandora's box open to all winds: anyone can accuse someone else of the worst misdeeds and vice versa, since every identitarian position is experienced as persecution.
>
> *(Roudinesco, 2022, p. 126–127)*

Signifiers such as "cultural appropriation" are precisely useful for understanding the narrow way that identity politics use diversity: the idea that one can "steal" the other's culture, or "take it," even if only in part, is based on the idea that one is the *possessor* of a culture, of an identity, for I can only appropriate 'illegitimately' the culture the other has/is. And it is this logic that sustains an identity understood as persecution: I am persecuted for being X. Following these lines, it should be clear to us why Roudinesco finds sad and strong connections between the discourses of political correctness, especially in its vein of 'woke canceling culture,' with the rise of the alt-right: both go down the same road of presumption of a total identity, they are not in obvious opposition but part of the same "line of an obscurantist counterrevolution" (p. 130), and both, 'woke' identity and the alt-right, "have made themselves advocates of a narcissism of small differences" (p. 136).[7]

It is because of this complicity with the satisfaction of the superego that all the movements of denunciation on social media, being preconditioned and overdetermined by the logic of sustaining the imago and the totalizing identity that these 'networks' construct, are always doomed to failure if their goal is to create a new social bond. Far from being able to build a collective and emancipating political force, they were trapped in the ability to judge others and to assume that the confession of one's own 'crimes' or the denunciation of the crimes of others were privileged ways to express our identity, but, in the end, "public confession does not constitute progress in itself" (Roudinesco, 2022, p. 19), and quite often, it leads to censorship, puritanism, the usurpation of the public powers by an individual.

The Imaginary deception offered by the politically correct activism of digital social media enthrones the narcissism of small differences, a classic Freudian theme, in the hypervigilance acts of censorship and puritanism such as demonstrating, through an etiquette, who I am:

> In other words, the #IamX is, above all, narcissistic: I am what I want, I want what I am, or even more succinctly, what I want to be. The volatile self functions as a floating signifier: it perseveres precisely because it floats, and it draws this function from its ephemeral condition. It is because of the internet and the digital that I can choose what I am: I am this or I am that; I am him or I am her; I just click it and I can be whatever I want! Isn't that the ultimate neoliberal message? You can be whatever you want, you just

> have to want it, just click it, you just have to buy this or that; and through this volatility you regain weight and materialize yourself (or should we say: incarnate yourself?). The #IamX becomes #Iam as such.
>
> *(De Vos, 2019, p. 48)*

The message offered in the neoliberal market of identities is not just about being what you want to be, but about being what you want to be *from among the options offered by the market*. It is what Renata Salecl (2010, p. 11) called "the tyranny of choice": the 'freedom' to choose is not chosen, the duty to choose has been imposed on us, which we must accept as proof of our freedom, so that it is in the choices I make that 'my' identity is reaffirmed. Neoliberalism uses marketing as a tool to 'detect' market niches, but, in reality, it has an interest in creating them: in making an identifying feature fashionable to which this or that product can be sold.[8]

This creation of niche markets is possible by the mechanisms of objectification of the subject, a culture that Lacan called "dominated as it is by objectifying ends" (1966, p. 96). What does it mean? What are the consequences, in the social bond, of a culture of objectification of the ego? Let's take a specific field that has benefited greatly from those objectifying ends to verify these consequences: labor psychology.

The servile ego (and its labor technification)

Why does psychoanalysis insist on attacking the ego? Freud put this at the center of the importance of the discovery of the unconscious, in his famous comparison with the Copernican revolution or Darwinian evolution (1955/XVII, pp. 139–141): while Copernicus dethroned our place in the center of the universe, and Darwin dethroned our place at the pinnacle of evolution, the unconscious dethrones the fortress of the ego.

Lacan emphasizes that the psychological discourses that deny this, or that try to give back to the ego the power it had lost, were involved in giving consistency to the imago: they wanted to help the ego to 'adapt' to its environment, to 'accept' reality. In these attempts, Lacan noted that the essential thing was to give the ego a supposed sense of individuality on the condition of making it *servile*:

> [I]t is clear that the promotion of the ego in our existence is leading, in conformity with the utilitarian conception of man that reinforces it, to an ever greater realization of man as an individual, in other words, in an isolation of the soul that is ever more akin to its original dereliction.
>
> *(Lacan, 1966, p. 99)*

The problem with this "realization of man as an individual," the promotion of the ego, is that it only occurs under the condition of a *quantification of* the ego, a *technification of the ego*, a subordination of the ego to a "utilitarian conception": the ego is only celebrated insofar as it can be measured, catalogued, explained—and exploited. This is why Lacan places the psychologization on the side of the machine:

> Correlatively, it seems [...] we are engaged in a technological enterprise on the scale of the entire species. The question is whether the conflict between Master and Slave will find its solution in the service of the machine, for which a psychotechnics, that is already yielding a rich harvest of ever more precise applications, will strive to provide race-car drivers and guards for regulating power stations.
>
> *(Lacan, 1966, p. 99)*

From this we extract another way of understanding psychologization: *psychotechnics at the service of the mechanization of the individual*. What Lacan warns of is how the reinforcement of the ego is the correlative of psychotechnics on the ego, a technical, utilitarian work on the ego. Any discourse that attempts to reinforce the ego through a psychologizing technique has the interest of turning the ego into a servant of the machine.

In a different text, *Presentation on Transference* (from 1951), Lacan presents this idea warning of the creation of a new alienation that is imposed in the relationship with reality, created "as much through the efforts of a collective belief as through the activity of selecting techniques with all the formative scope of rituals: in short, a *homo psychologicus*, the danger of which I am warning you against" (pp. 177–178). *Homo psychologicus* is a product of the working conditions in which he lives, which cause the problems that define him as such.

This becomes quite obvious in the psychotechnical neoliberalization of the field of psychology itself in what we know today as "labor psychology." This is nothing new; it is a phenomenon that has been systematically developed since the beginning of the last century in an attempt to create an "applied psychology." Hugo Münsterberg began his 1913 book *Psychology and Industrial Efficiency* as follows:

> Our aim is to sketch the outlines of a new science which is to intermediate between the modern laboratory psychology and the problems of economics: the psychological experiment is systematically to be placed at the service of commerce and industry.
>
> *(Münsterberg, [1913] 2012)*

If we follow Matthew Hale Jr. (1980, p. 149), Münsterberg's interest was in the creation of a psychology that saw the management of the labor force as something as important as the management of the machinery of production. For Hale Jr. (pp. 149–150), the basis of this interest lay in the Taylorist system of work standardization, of providing individual incentives to workers instead of a collective discussion of their working conditions, and creating a 'scientific' way to manage workers in an industry. What Münsterberg wanted from psychology was to find the means to take control of deciding the *best* way to manage that workforce, regardless of the empirical knowledge of the factory owners and, obviously, the interests of the workers. As a good technocratic positivist, what Münsterberg yearned for was the hyperscientification of life, in this case specifically (for he was interested in many areas of social life), working life.

What was at the basis of this hypertechnified psychologization of working life? The *measurement* of individual labor power, the possibility that each individual at work could be *measured and classified* with the aim of making them more productive. This classification was soon sustained in the interest of studying the "mental types" of each worker in order to assign them the task that "best suits" their mental type. In the conclusions of his book, Münsterberg cites the experiment of a sociologist who sent thousands of questionnaires to workers in all kinds of factories and then classified their responses into "mental types," thus managing to account for variables of the working conditions, from fatigue to satisfaction with the salary received. From this experiment, "[m]any psychological elements of industrial life thus come to a sharp focus and the strong individual differences could not be brought out in a more characteristic way" (Münsterberg, [1913] 2012).

The legacy of these ideas is a treatise such as that of J.A.C. Brown (1954), which presents arguments in favor of the application of the principles of psychology in the workplace, and in particular in each of its strata: the importance and advantages of "opinion surveys" (pp. 172–173), techniques to disguise labor hierarchies by making managers 'behave like' the workers (p. 196) and recommendations to have "democratic methods of control" (p 232). In these examples, we verify how Münsterberg's individualized classification project mutated into the implementation of techniques and standards of behavior control at work, imposed from psychology onto managers and workers.

Communication studies didn't hesitate in quickly adopting these imperatives of technical management of the work force. The favorite arm of this is the so-called "organizational communication," a discipline interested in offering techniques to 'enable' communication, specifically, 'assertive communication.' In her book on this topic, Anni Townend comes to trust so blindly in the magic power of words[9] that she even asks not to use certain pronouns so that one is "one's own person":

> When people use the personal pronoun "I" rather than "You," "We," "One," or "It," they communicate much more powerfully a sense of self, and of taking responsibility for their feelings, thoughts, and behavior. It can sometimes be difficult for people who are used to saying "You," "We," or "One," to use "I." When they do, they notice a qualitative

> difference in both how they communicate and what they are communicating, and the impact that they have on others. In particular they have a much stronger sense of self, of being their own person.
>
> *(Townend, 2007, p. 39)*

What the Lacanian mirror stage warns against is precisely not believing that I am my "own person" just because I avoid conjugating verbs with certain grammatical persons. These kinds of practices, which flood business manuals, are based on a certain naive *coaching* that pretends, as Townend herself asks us (p. 31), that we "take risks," that we "trust," that we "make mistakes." What kind of I is it that these kinds of ideas propose, if not an I that is always in harmony with itself, that disavows that constitutive split of its own subjectivity, that believes it is the 'owner' of the language it uses? It is difficult to understand why a person who "is used" to saying "you" instead of "I" has "a much stronger sense of self": is that evident in the number of times they conjugate their verbs in one way or another? It seems that the Greek maxim of "know thyself" is now reduced to the number of verb conjugations or the use of personal pronouns.[10]

It is because of this type of idea that Lacan, in *The Mirror Stage*, mistrusts philosophy that is committed to full consciousness, to 'knowing oneself,' or to discourses that promote being the master of one's own destiny, that promote "a self-sufficiency of consciousness, [...] the illusion of autonomy" (1966, p. 80). What the mirror stage shows is that what one believes about oneself *is a deception*: any philosophy that advocates full consciousness, a subject that *knows itself*, is exactly the opposite of what psychoanalytic experience shows, which, before assuming the ego as the axis of knowledge of reality, starts rather from the "*function of misrecognition*" (p. 80) that characterizes the ego, from the fact that in the ego there is something that operates on the margins and against its will.

In today's companies, communication departments tend to work closely with human resources departments, whose very name reveals their interest: to treat humans as another resource for the company's profits. The neoliberalization of labor is evidenced by the fact that these departments proliferate even beyond what, if we were naive enough, we would not call companies: public universities, hospitals, bureaucratic offices, civil society organizations also have their human resources. The psychologists who feed the operating manuals of these departments, who are no longer called "industrial psychologists" but "labor psychologists," are based on the behaviorist results of written tests, which have the explicit interest of reducing human subjectivity to quantitative data, of how many times the subject has felt "sad" or "motivated" at work, to mention an example from my personal experience as a worker in a company, so that they can be 'managed' properly.

Criticism of this type of practice has been circulating for several decades. A special place is occupied by Maurice de Montmollin's book *Les psychopitres* (1972; *The psychoclowns* could be the translation). This book has a certain value as a critique because its author devoted himself to occupational psychology for several years, and he recognizes how signifiers such as "initiative," "intuition," "adaptability" and "team spirit" permeate what the labor psychologist looks for when searching for the best "candidate," a practice done, supposedly, through tests and measurements "more precise, more modern and more scientific" (p. 10).

We should not underestimate Montmollin's critique as part of the fashion for critical readings of the 1960s and 1970s. In a more contemporary work, Luis Enrique Alonso and Carlos Fernández Rodríguez (2018) have clearly shown how this type of conceptualization of what workers *are*, although we can find its origins in the intellectual atmosphere Münsterberg worked in, has its most important antecedent in the economic neoliberalization that took place most intensely and systematically during the 1980s, when the end of the European and North American welfare states receded from public discourse on economy, leaving the business classes to dictate what effectively became economic policies. And as should be obvious by now, these different economic conditions have an impact on subjectivity, making it clear that neoliberalism is not simply an economic model, but a mode of social bond. With its ability to weaken the sense of community, entrenched in a "*managerial thinking*" full of mechanistic metaphors of social life, neoliberalism no longer has any interest in concealing the conditions of exploitation in which people will work: 'willingness to work in a team,''working by goals,' 'ease of communication,' 'tolerance to frustration,' 'proactivity and initiative,' among other generic formulations, are what we come across today when reading job descriptions on digital platforms (whether to be a sales manager in a branch, to work in office administration or to teach university courses).

The drawn self (and its process of drawing)

Some of the common methods used by "human resources" departments to select candidates are the "person in the rain" and "draw an animal" tests. The point of these tests is that the candidate complies with the instruction to draw what the test is called, and then adds details such as the story of that "person" or that "animal." These tests are not simply a creative digression in a job interview, but rather they aim to show the person's ability to perform a job based on a series of parameters that, when we approach the methodology to study them, are quite contradictory. For example, in the ways Graciela Celener (2006, pp. 123–129) explains how to interpret the results are far from clear: it is good that the candidates have provided enough details in the "person in the rain" (to demonstrate that they can specialize, that they have "analytical thinking", p. 123), but it is not good to include too many details (to show that he/she can adapt to different tasks, that he/she has "synthetic" thinking, p. 123); if the candidate concentrated on drawing the person from the waist up, that's indicative of "conventional thinking" and "practical judgment" (p. 124), but it is also good if the person is drawn in full length, for that shows the candidate has great "empathy" (p. 126). These parameters are paradoxical, and it is impossible to find a drawing that shows as many positive as negative indicators.

With these types of tests, the more we can adapt the resulting drawing to established models on how to read it, the more we demonstrate that the test shows us the subject's aptitude for work: the interpretation of the drawing serves to demonstrate the validity of the parameter for its interpretation. It is a tautological argument that, today, appears to have great dimensions of objectivity in "labor psychology." There have been some critiques of these tests (e.g., the argument from Imuta, Scarf, Pharo & Hayne (2013), who advocate against considering them a way to 'demonstrate' intelligence), but versions of them are still quite popular in many processes for job applicants.

Curiously, psychoanalysis has also taken an interest in children's drawings. Unlike the psychologizing practices that verify the drawing as a product to be analyzed, the drawing is understood psychoanalytically as a process in itself. The difference between these two positions is that the drawing itself is not as important as the process in which it is drawn, so that it is always anchored in the drawer. That's why Marisa Rodulfo (2016) considers such drawing-as-process as similar to the Freudian dream work: more than the final drawing, it is as important when the children or persons doing them turn the page, change the pencil or color, or what they say when they are drawing it.

And now we go back to Lacan. When he pointed out that the strengthening of the ego has the consequence of "an ever greater realization of man as an individual" (1966, p. 99), he was referring to the fact that our social bond in a psychologized world, where psychology is psychotechnics at the service of the machine, is based on a correspondence between the ego and the individual that psychology accounts for with its standardized measurements. The objective of these measurements, of all that advice on assertiveness and the procurement of good leadership at work, is to deny the experience of the constitutive split of subjectivity, so that labor psychology, with its instruments, is able to tell me what I am: measuring me and offering me the result of its tests as 'objective' evidence of what I 'really' am.

While the Lacanian mirror stage places a split at the birth of human subjectivity, a split that does not allow the ego to be at peace with its own self and body due to the subject, psychologization consists of exactly the opposite: by strengthening the ego by disavowing the distance between its self and its body, by providing the mechanisms to deny the existence of the subject, by establishing the coordinates to tell the ego *what it is.*

The labor psychologist leaves aside the study of the psyche in order to "to provide race-car drivers and guards for regulating power stations" (Lacan, 1966, p. 99), so that the singularities of each worker and their universal conditions of exploitation do not matter: the essential thing is that they are, according to pre-designed tests, the best candidate/race-car driver/guard for this or that position.

This offers yet another way of understanding psychologization: *the creation of a narrative of an individual that can be completely and objectively measured and studied*, via the universal measurement of psychological tests. The mantra of psychology when it shows us the results of the tests and their interpretations, which have the explicit interest of characterizing subjectivity in pre-written 'mental types,' is "*You are that.*" The greatest triumph of psychologization is to erase the distance between the individual and the category that explains it: the category doesn't explain my behavior, but *I am that category.* When labor psychology classifies me, it is not only telling me what I am, but *demonstrating* what I am: the description of my subjectivity has the effects of creating my subjectivity. Psychologization inhabits, and disavows, the threshold where the other's desire becomes my desire, where the identity offered to me by the other is the identity I choose, where the other's imperative "*You are that*" becomes "*I am that.*"

Notes

1 Prior even to the more famous one found in the *Seminar on "The Purloined Letter"* (1966, p. 30): "in which the sender, as I tell you, receives from the receiver his own message in an inverted form."
2 As we will see later, for Roudinesco—and I ascribe to this idea as well—it is very pernicious, or at least ignorant, to describe the 'woke' movement as 'leftist'. There is nothing inherently 'leftist' in using a different pronoun when referring to someone, or to denounce macho violence on social media, which is a trap that many people, both those who defend such 'affirmative' actions and those who detest them, fall for, due to ignorance of history and complexities of the left, or due to the perverse superego logic that sustains them.
3 Again, Jan de Vos's *Psychologization and the Subject of Late Modernity* (2013) is particularly clarifying here.
4 Of course, we can find many examples in language: it was only when I started talking frequently with Mexicans who were not from the part of Mexico where I grew up (Yucatan) that I became aware of many words, turns of phrases and accents we have in my region of origin: it was only when my particular Mexican 'identity' couldn't be grounded in reality (i.e., it was not total) that I stumbled upon its incompleteness; and, further, this experience of 'having' an identity was even more shackled when, coming back to Yucatan after spending months in Mexico City, my friends mocked my Mexico City accent, whereas my contacts in Mexico City always mocked my Yucatecan accent. Again, in the terrains of food, I guess readers from Venezuela and Colombia might think of a similar example with the arepa: the first time I had it, I was with a Venezuelan friend, who complained that "this is not a *true* arepa." The Venezuelan identity, for her, was in the stone that disturbed the access to the 'true' Venezuelan arepa (a sort of Lacanian *agalma*, perhaps?).
5 This is a basic tenet of Marxism: the main objective of all consumption is to sustain production, so that in capitalism one does not produce in order to consume (as 'common' sense would have it), but rather one consumes in order that production may continue (see Marx [1857] 1973, p. 91).

6 It might be interesting to connect this with the idea of animal and human deceptions in the chapter dedicated to animals and Lacan.

7 Despite this apparent ostracizing, radical criticism, Roudinesco comments that we can establish a certain distinction between 'woke culture' vs. the alt- and far-right: unlike wokeness, on the right "no awakening is possible" (p. 138), in the sense that the far-right (and religious ultra-fundamentalism too) is sustained by the narrative of a return to a glorious origin that is being destroyed or has been destroyed by the foreigner, the stranger, the alien. In a way, 'woke culture' tells us how *the world we live in is not so innocent* because it is riddled with almost imperceptible identity struggles (as evidenced by ideas such as 'micromachismos'), while the far-right tells us how the world we live in *is a perversion of a 'normal' world*, if not the remains after the destruction brought about by having allowed otherness into our territories. What they both share, then, is the pretense of elevating identity in a hierarchy *sustained by the ego and its image (i.e., it(s)self)*; and what they both cannot do is a universal and emancipatory politics sustained in the division of the subject.

8 As has been shown on many occasions, this is not strange even in matters that one would believe to be 'objective' and unrelated to commercial interests such as health: indeed, even diseases are created and sustained in order to create a market niche. As has now become quite obvious, the fentanyl crisis in North America was produced precisely by the freedom pharmaceutical companies have to produce drugs for aches that didn't need it in the first place: it created a solution in order to create a problem; they created their own niche market (addicts of their own drugs) for those to whom they sell their products (to help them overcome their addiction). See an introduction to this issue here: www.npr.org/2023/05/26/1178372700/dea-morris-dickson-drug-distributor-license-opioid-crisis.

9 It is worth remembering that, in *Totem and Taboo*, Freud indicates (1958/XIII, p. 56) that a classic feature of psychic infantilism and primitive civilizations is the belief that words have a magical power that is invoked when they are used.

10 Francisco Clavijo Tapia and Uriel Bustamante Lozano (2019) applied these same Townend's principles to the study of organizational discourse in an enterprise. Among their conclusions is that bosses hold employees responsible for the challenges of the company when speaking in second person plural sentences, so that "employees are firstly recognized" (p. 282); however, employees "do not accept responsibility for their actions" (p. 282). One cannot help but wonder why employees are so irresponsible with such assertive bosses who communicate in the first person. Again, one also wonders what kind of "I" organizational communication studies are talking about when they ask us to communicate 'assertively.' Are they that naive, or do they think we are?

References

Brown, J. A. C. (1954). *The Social Psychology of Industry. Human Relations in the Factory.* Penguin Books.

Celener, Graciela. (2006). "Indicadores de las competencias psicológicas del perfil del puesto desde las técnicas proyectivas gráficas". In Graciela Celener (ed.). *Técnicas proyectivas. Actualización e interpretación en los ámbitos clínico, laboral y forense. Tomo II*, pp. 121–134. Lugar Editorial.

Clavijo Tapia, Francisco Javier & Bustamante Lozano, Uriel. (2019). "Comunicación asertiva y productiva: Caso de estudio en Manizales". *NOVUM. Revista de Ciencias Sociales Aplicadas*, Vol. 1, No. 9, pp. 261–285.

De Montmollin, Maurice. (1972). *Les psychopitres: une autocritique de la psychologie industrielle.* Presses Universitaires de France.

De Vos, Jan. (2013). *Psychologization and the Subject of Late Modernity.* Palgrave Macmillan.
De Vos, Jan. (2019). *La psicologización y sus vicisitudes.* Paradiso.
Debord, Guy. [1967] (1995). *The Society of the Spectacle.* (Translated Donald Nicholson-Smith). Zone Books.
Enrique Alonso, Luis & Fernández Rodríguez, Carlos J. (2018). *Poder y sacrificio. Los nuevos discursos de la empresa.* Siglo XXI (epub).
Freud, Sigmund. [1895] (1966). "Project For a Scientific Psychology". In *The Standard Edition of The Complete Psychological Works of Sigmund Freud*, Vol. I. The Hogarth Press, pp. 281–397.
Freud, Sigmund. [1913] (1958). "Totem and Taboo". In *The Standard Edition of The Complete Psychological Works of Sigmund Freud*, Vol. XIII. The Hogarth Press, pp. 1–162.
Freud, Sigmund. [1917] (1955). "A Difficulty in the Path of Psycho-Analysis". In *The Standard Edition of The Complete Psychological Works of Sigmund Freud*, Vol. XVII. The Hogarth Press, pp. 135–144.
Freud, Sigmund. [1921] (1955). "Group Psychology and the Analysis of the Ego". In *The Standard Edition of The Complete Psychological Works of Sigmund Freud*, Vol. XVIII. The Hogarth Press, pp. 65–143.
HaleJr., Matthew. (1980). *Human science and social order. Hugo Münsterberg and the Origins of Applied Psychology.* Temple University Press.
Imuta, Kana, Scarf, Damian, Pharo, Henry & Hayne, Harlene. (2013). "Drawing a close to the use of human figure drawings as a projective measure of intelligence." *PLoS ONE*, 8 (3): e58991, 8 pgs.
Lacan, Jacques. [1936] (2006). "Beyond the 'Reality Principle'." In *Écrits. The First Complete Edition in English.* W.W. Norton & Company, pp. 58–74.
Lacan, Jacques. [1948] (2006). "Aggressiveness in Psychoanalysis." In *Écrits. The First Complete Edition in English.* W.W. Norton & Company, pp. 82–101.
Lacan, Jacques. [1949] (2006). "The Mirror Stage as Formative of the *I* Function as Revealed in Psychoanalytic Experience." In *Écrits. The First Complete Edition in English.* W.W. Norton & Company, pp. 75–81.
Lacan, Jacques. [1950] (2006). "A Theoretical Introduction to the Functions of Psychoanalysis in Criminology." In *Écrits. The First Complete Edition in English.* W.W. Norton & Company, pp. 102–122.
Lacan, Jacques. [1951] (2006). "Presentation on Transference." In *Écrits. The First Complete Edition in English.* W.W. Norton & Company, pp. 176–185.
Lacan, Jacques. [1953–1954] (1988). *The Seminar of Jacques Lacan. Book I. Freud's Papers on Technique.* W.W. Norton & Company.
Lacan, Jacques. [1956] (2006). "Seminar on 'The Purloined Letter'." In *Écrits. The First Complete Edition in English.* W.W. Norton & Company, pp. 6–57.
Lacan, Jacques. [1956] (2006). "The Situation of Psychoanalysis and the Training of Psychoanalysts in 1956." In *Écrits. The First Complete Edition in English.* W.W. Norton & Company, pp. 384–407.
Lacan, Jacques. [1960] (2006). "Remarks on Daniel Lagache's Presentation: 'Psychoanalysis and Personality Structure'." In *Écrits. The First Complete Edition in English.* W.W. Norton & Company, pp. 543–574.
Marx, Karl. [1857–1858] (1973). *Grundrisse: Foundations of the Critique of Political Economy (Rough Draft).* (Translated with a Foreword by Martin Nicolaus). Penguin Books, New Left Review.
Münsterberg, Hugo. [1913] (2012). *Psychology and Industrial Efficiency.* Duke Classics (epub).

Pavón-Cuéllar, David & Capulín Arellano, María Concepción Lizeth. (2023). "Ocho aportes del marximo y del psicoanálisis para una radicalización del enfoque interseccional." *Memoria, Revista de crítica militante*, No. 286, pp. 70–75.

Rodulfo, Marisa. (2016). *El niño del dibujo.* Paidós.

Roudinesco, Elisabeth. [2021] (2022). *The Sovereign Self. Pitfalls of Identity Politics.* Polity.

Salecl, Renata. (2010). *Choice.* Profile Books.

Townend, Anni. (2007). *Assertiveness and Diversity.* Palgrave Macmillan.

Žižek, Slavoj. (2018). *Like a Thief in Broad Daylight: Power in the Era of Post-Human Capitalism.* Seven Stories Press.

7

CONCLUDING REMARKS

You are that Manticore

The Lacanian mirror stage offers us a conception of the development of human subjectivity as something that is traversed by the other from its very emergence—that is, the very figure of the ego *necessarily* presupposes the other. This traversing of the ego by the other leaves as a consequence an inherent imbalance in the ego, a split ego, an imbalance evident in the relationship with its own body (which is experienced as alien, as having a will of its own), in the relationship with its own image (which is experienced as something that seems of its own but is always at the service and scrutiny of the other) and in the emergence of the *subject*, that residue that remains once the self is alienated in its image. The subject supposes that which hinders the totalization of the ego, which hinders the omnipotence of the imago, which destroys the empire of the self. In a way, psychologizing practices and the neoliberal marketing share the common task of disavowing the split ego in order to erect an empire of the self.

The mirror stage also offers three consequences to understand the nature of human subjectivity: (1) the human subject, with its inherent split, ends up far from any 'natural animality'; (2) aggressiveness towards others, far from being a pathological issue, is a necessary step for the construction of one's own subjectivity; and (3) what the ego experiences as its own desire is, in reality, an alienation to the desire of the other (both to desire what the other desires and to desire to be the object that the other desires).

We traversed these consequences of the mirror stage in a previous discussion on the importance of the Freudian concept of identification (both as a moment in transference and as a mental infection), as it is a key part in the Lacanian conception of the mirror stage. And through the exposition, we verified certain problems present in some mainstream readings about our animal condition, relation to digital images and identity policies. We

DOI: 10.4324/9781003640653-7

stumbled upon a Lacanian reading of deception in the animal world, the problems in zoology's attempts to inquire into animal cognition, and the radical alienation from/within our world when we try to look at animals. We also found the deficiencies of some mainstream reading of the idea of selfie present in communication and media studies, and the ways the selfie enforces an illusion of ownership of 'our own' images, with the problematic consequences this illusion carries (as exposed in revenge-porn pictures). Finally, we took a reflection on how this sense of 'empowering the ego,' through the celebration of the self, functions quite appropriately for an economic system, neoliberalism, that argues for dismantling any collective form of emancipation and for enforcing a hyperindividualism.

To approach the ending of our journey, let's return to the Lacanian text to have a final reflection on a strange phrase there:

> In the subject to subject recourse we preserve, psychoanalysis can accompany the patient to the ecstatic limit of the "*Thou art that*," where the cipher of his mortal destiny is revealed to him, but it is not in our sole power as practitioners to bring him to the point where the true journey begins.
>
> *(Lacan, 1966, p. 82)*

That phrase "Thou art that," "You are that," is undoubtedly something that appears in many places that psychologize the ego, as we saw in the previous chapter, in order to elude the subject. So, what is the "you are that" that Lacan talks about?

You, are, that

This mirror stage aphorism, "You are that," can open three different readings.

First, we can read an *objectifying description* in "You are *that*": the subject is told that *it is that thing* that is being shown to them. The result of a brain scan, the result of a personality test, the diagnosis thrown up by manuals such as the DSM, the psychiatrizing diagnosis: what operates here is a discourse completely oblivious to the singular enunciation of the subject, a discourse only interested in the diagnostic manuals and the results established by the machine, a discourse that takes the subject as *an object to be scientifically described.*

Second, we could read a *subjective assumption* in "*You* are that": the subject *assumes it(s)self* in what is shown to it. This second reading starts moving away from the positivism of the previous one, for it is no longer just about what is shown to the subject, but about the assumption the subject takes in what is being shown, an identification with what the other shows to the subject. However, this could still be not enough, because in today's hyperdiagnosed world, we constantly find what Freud called, in his Lecture XXIV, "[taking] flight into illness [...] 'gain from illness'" (1963/XVI, pp. 382–383). Psychologizing discourses have a lot of power and scope to explain my/self and my behaviors, but I can relate to those explanations alienated from any subjective assumption of them, as a knowledge that produces no subjective implications for me. It is quite common, in the psychoanalytic clinic, to listen to people who start their psychoanalytic process listing all the diagnoses that psychologists, psychiatrists, therapists and even coaches have given them before, desperate because they do not understand *why* they cannot change even though *they know what they have.*

Finally, in a dialectical inversion, we have a *subjectifying description/objective assumption* in "*You* are *that*": instead of thinking "*that*" as the result of the test/diagnosis, we could think of the *that* of which psychoanalysis speaks and that Lacan wrote as *ça*, and instead of thinking "You" as the 'transparent' ego with 'inherent' qualities, we could think of the split subject Lacan based his teaching on. *You are that, that* which is symptomatic, enigmatic, nonsensical to the ego in *you.*

For example, the analysand who arrives at her first session saying that, after years with psychologists and psychiatrists, and having had various diagnoses and therapies, she *doesn't understand why nothing changes*: here the issue is not whether the diagnoses were *correct or not* (that would be the first reading), or whether the patient *really* understood them or believes in them (that would be the second reading); here the issue is *the question itself*, not how to answer it from knowledge but how to accommodate it as a question, to open a space for such question to exert consequences in the subject. The diagnosis is understood, *one knows one('s)self*, but there is something that operates against meaning, against knowledge, against consciousness, against understanding, that causes that *question*: why am I the way I am, even though I know what I am? It is a description of something that is not only subjective but singular, something that is unknown even to my/self, that operates unconsciously, where I find my subjectivity as an object upon which this "*that*" operates.

When I talked about the description of the identity of the job applicant in the so-called "projective tests" of labor psychology, we noted a good example of an *objectifying description* in the fact that if the person under the rain was holding or not an umbrella, *that means X or Y*; and we noted a good example of a *subjective assumption* in the fact that, when the labor psychologist reads to the applicant from a manual the meaning of her/his drawing, the applicant *identifies with the explanation*, expressing 'yes, that's me!'

However, couldn't a drawing of my/self, made by the other, become an external point that *draws*, that extracts, from an interiority that I can't simply recognize as my/self?

A monster with a human face

The Spanish film *Mantícora* (dir. Carlos Vermut, 2022) has a scene where this is explicitly staged. The film tells the story of Julián, a young man who rescues a boy, Cristian, from a fire, and after this heroic act, he begins to have pedophilic desires towards the child. Julián works in a videogames company, designing digital avatars of monsters for an upcoming release. Using this technology and expertise, he designs an avatar of the child that he can see and manipulate through his virtual-reality headset. Feeling somewhat regretful about the whole situation, he deletes the avatar file, moves from the apartment building and starts a romantic relationship with a woman, Diana. Throughout the film, it is very clear that Julián feels these pedophilic desires not only as something to be hidden from others but also as something that he himself tries to fight against by hiding it, a desire that he recognizes as his own, but one that he cannot take hold of or control and tries to extirpate. It is as if rather than Julián having a pedophilic desire, *it is the pedophilic desire that owns Julián*. However, after discovering the child avatar, his company fires him, the news gets to Diana who dumps him (telling him she is disgusted by this whole idea), and on the brink of desperation, Julián gives in to this desire he had tried to keep out of his life and goes to Cristian's house with the clear intention of raping him.

Just before doing so, with the child drugged and in bed, Julián notices a drawing that Cristian made about a fantasy Julián confessed to him on the day of the fire: that, as a child, he wanted "to be a tiger." The drawing is of a tiger with a human head—hence the title of the film—which, upon seeing it on the wall, prevents Julián from continuing what he was about to do, and he decides to throw himself out of the window.

The first reading we could make of this scene is that Julián saw himself 'as a monster,' because of the act he planned and was about to carry out; feeling guilty, he decides to atone for the sin by committing suicide. This reading, although not entirely a misfire, leaves out something essential: it is through an image offered by the other that Julián becomes aware of him/self and of his act; that is, once again we are presented with the way out of the psychologization by recognizing that the subject's act cannot fail to pass through the other. Julián came across an image made by the other person (an objectifying description of his childhood fantasy) which he subjectively assumed as his, and which points to something alien to Julián's interiority: his desire for something he desires not to desire.

The following scene complements and arrives at another understanding of what Julián (and the subject) is for the other. We realize that it was a failed suicide, and the protagonist has ended up paralyzed for life. In the hospital bed, due to the multiple surgeries, he must lie face down, and they put a mirror on the floor so that he can see the people who come to visit him and stand behind his back. The doctor (with whom he interacts through the mirror) arrives and explains the situation, and announces a visitor: it is Diana, his former girlfriend, who begins to talk to him through the mirror, but she soon decides to stand in front of him, on the floor. With this act, she proves to be the only person who, even if she doesn't *understand* or approve of his intention for the act he was about to commit, offers him *her* face as the condition of the possibilities of a bond that no one else has offered him. While Julián verifies what he *is* in the image given by the other (the drawing, the words spoken to him at the company after the discovery), Diana allows him to leave the circuit of the image by offering him her face (and not the image of her face in the mirror).

In other words: she offers him the possibility to surpass the circuit of the image and let him confront the face of the other. It is in front of the face of the other, in the other's presence, and not in the image of the other, where the subject confronts the point of impossibility of its own totality; it is only against the face of the other that I can find my own incompleteness, as the biblical quote, quite apt for this scene, tells us: "Now we see in a mirror dimly, but then face to face. Now I know in part, but then I shall know just as I also am known" (1 Corinthians 13:12, New International Version[1]).

The face of Diana, the face of the other, presents Julián with the possibility of, finally, confronting his own desire, but not in the simplistic idea of 'coming to terms with it' (the film never states, clearly, what the future holds for Julián), nor 'to atone his own sin' (the film is not a moralizing pamphlet[2]), but to open the space for a subjectivity, his own subjectivity, as something that cannot be totally known, totally transparent: the final scene, where Diana tells him about a movie where a man discovers a room in his house he had never seen before, almost explicitly points to the idea that there is something deep within ourselves which is, precisely because of that, foreign to us. *Mantícora* uses a desire that is so taboo to show us how, as such, *all our desire is foreign to us since it comes from (the place of) the other*: we should not think of desire as something that emanates directly from us, as something inherent in our mind or genetic code and over which we have omnipotent control, but rather as something that escapes our will, as something that imposes not only a desire for something but a desire for desire itself.

Where the true journey begins

To conclude, the recognition of that which is *an otherness in my desire* offers us the reasons why a psychoanalysis cannot be carried out from outside the subject's involvement in it: one cannot 'psychoanalyze' someone who does not undertake an analysis voluntarily (e.g., by court order or from psychiatric confinement), or who does not submit to the fundamental rule of psychoanalysis. This is why Lacan indicates that it is not only in the power of the analyst to bring the subject "to the point where the true journey begins" (p. 82).

Where does the journey begin? It is incorrect to say that it begins only in the ego, because it begins in the recognition of that which is *an otherness in the* ego, that which operates *on the margins* of the ego, that which seems to be *less and more* than the ego at the same time, that which is not my body and is my body *at the same time*, that which is *inhuman* because it is *too* human, that which is *fragmentary* and at the same time *totalizing*, that which is *my desire* and at the same time *the desire of the other… that* which *I* am.

Notes

1 See here: www.biblegateway.com/passage/?search=1Cor.13.12&version=NIV
2 In case it is necessary, as I have found out in some places discussing this film, I should also mention that the fact that the film is not *about* punishing someone with pedophilic desires does not mean that the film celebrates, justifies or minimizes them. Having been a lecturer on film courses for years, I have realized how often students (of all ages and from all places) fall into the trap of believing that because a film deals with pedophilia (or any other disturbing or complex topic) and does not explicitly condemn it, *therefore* it condones it or makes a case for it. This naive reading of *Manticora* makes us lose the point the film is trying to make.

References

Freud, Sigmund. [1917] (1963). "Lecture XXIV: The Common Neurotic State." In *The Standard Edition of The Complete Psychological Works of Sigmund Freud*, Vol. XVI. The Hogarth Press, pp. 378–391.
Lacan, Jacques. [1949] (2006). "The Mirror Stage as Formative of the *I* Function as Revealed in Psychoanalytic Experience." In *Écrits. The First Complete Edition in English*. W.W. Norton & Company, pp. 75–81.

INDEX

For Product Safety Concerns and Information please contact our EU representative GPSR@taylorandfrancis.com
Taylor & Francis Verlag GmbH, Kaufingerstraße 24, 80331 München, Germany

www.ingramcontent.com/pod-product-compliance
Ingram Content Group UK Ltd.
Pitfield, Milton Keynes, MK11 3LW, UK
UKHW022359190926
475702UK00015B/2386
9781041074663